ALSO BY SUE FLEMING

Buff Brides

Buff Moms-to-Be

BUFF MOMS

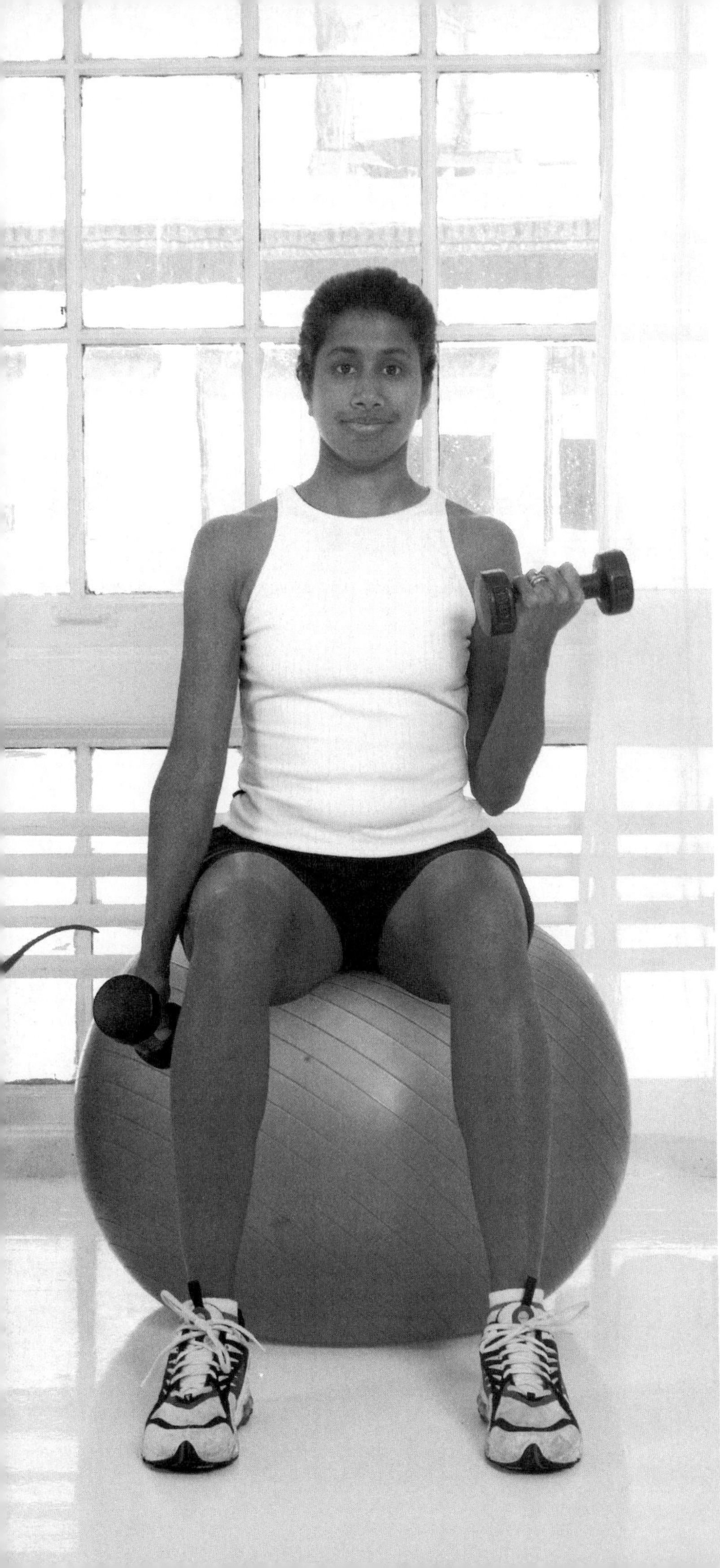

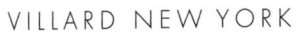

VILLARD NEW YORK

BUFF MOMS

MOMS

The Complete
Guide to
Fitness for
All Mothers

Sue Fleming

LIBRARY OF CONGRESS CATALOGING-IN-PUBLICATION DATA

Fleming, Sue
Buff moms: the complete guide to fitness for all mothers/Sue Fleming.
p.   cm.
ISBN 0-8129-7224-4 (pbk.)
1. Postnatal care. 2. Physical fitness for women. 3. Exercise for women.
4. Mothers—Health and hygiene. I. Title.

RG801.F56 2004
613.7'045—dc22   2004053566

Villard Books website address: www.villard.com

Printed in the United States of America

9 8 7 6 5 4 3 2 1

First Edition

Book design by Mary A. Wirth

I dedicate this book to all those who listened,
all those who helped me find my dreams,
all those who cared.

And to Mom, who doesn't have to suffer anymore.

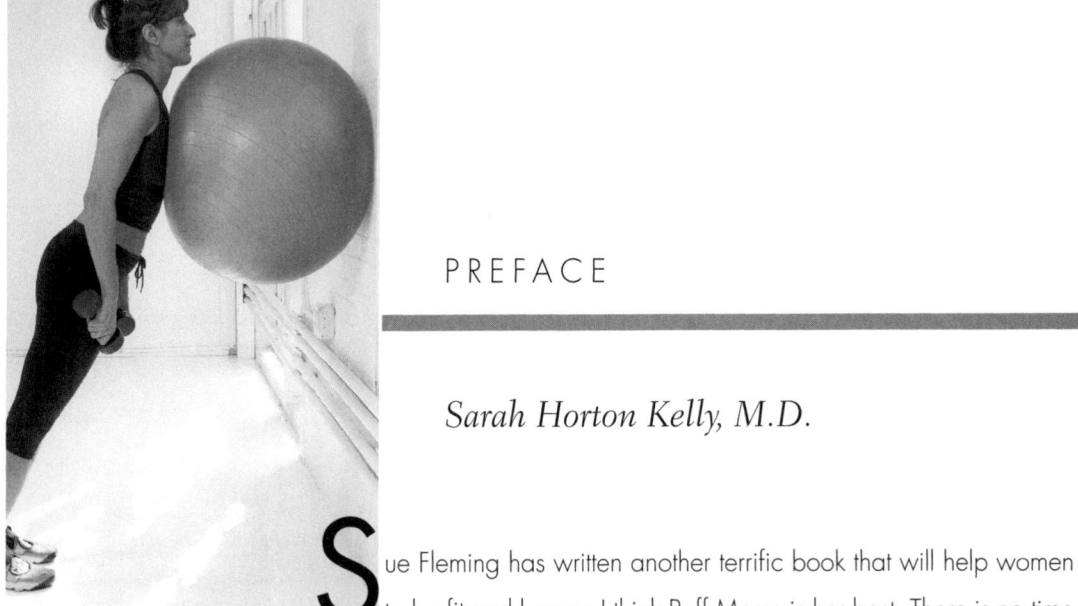

PREFACE

Sarah Horton Kelly, M.D.

S ue Fleming has written another terrific book that will help women to be fit and happy. I think Buff Moms is her best. There is no time in a woman's life as difficult and challenging as when she brings home a new baby. Plummeting hormone levels, family stresses, erratic sleep, and a body changing into something that she may not like, all contribute to making the postpartum mother at risk for anxiety and depression. A new mother recovering from a cesarean section or a difficult vaginal delivery may suffer additional pain and fatigue. A nursing mother must adjust to breast changes, possibly to discomfort, and to the responsibility of being the source of nourishment for her baby. If she is a first-time mother, she must learn how to care for her child and develop the mothering skills that will foster the growth of her baby. Likewise, if she is bringing her baby home to a household with other children, she has to face the challenges of caring for her older children as well as meeting the twenty-four-hour demands of her new baby. Obviously, the postpartum period is not an easy time, nevertheless it is usually a time of incredible joy and love.

This book gives excellent advice and teaches skills that will guide new mothers through this stressful time. Exercise is extremely beneficial for the new mom. As she starts a program for weight loss and body strengthening and toning, she begins to feel better physically, mentally, and emotionally. Exercise alone has been shown to decrease depression in post-partum women. By devoting time to herself and her concerns, a new mom gains perspective on her life and role. She is refreshed by working out and is able to give more focused care to her baby.

The American College of Obstetricians and Gynecologists (ACOG) teaches that the postpartum body slowly returns to its normal state over six to eight weeks. A gradual resumption of physical activity to pre-pregnancy levels is considered safe. ACOG now emphasizes that physical exercise is very beneficial for all women. They explain that moderate weight loss while nursing is safe for the baby and will not affect its growth. They advise women who have had a cesarean to avoid physical activity that could strain their abdominal walls, since their tissues have been weakened and need extra time to heal. However, they can walk, do some exercises, and by eight weeks postpartum start routines that strengthen their abdominal-wall muscles. ACOG also warns mothers not to breast-feed their infants immediately after exercising, since the lactic acid produced by exercising muscles can cause breast milk to taste bitter, possibly dissuading babies from nursing.

I want to praise Sue for her work. She has a rare gift for inspiring even the busiest "I don't have time" mom onto the exercise mat and on to physical fitness. Her exercises are simple and easy to perform. Sue gives the terrific suggestion that you take, at the least, ten minutes a day to do an exercise routine. This is doable by virtually every mom and gives significant benefits over time. In several weeks you will improve your body tone, stamina, and sense of well-being.

Sue intersperses excellent advice on dieting, nutrition, and physical training throughout her book. I suggest that you start by quickly reading the entire book. Then go back, set goals for yourself, and outline an exercise program for the next month.

Finally, remember that exercise feels good—and makes you feel better.

Sarah Horton Kelly, M.D.
Obstetrician and Gynecologist
Columbia University College of
Physicians and Surgeons

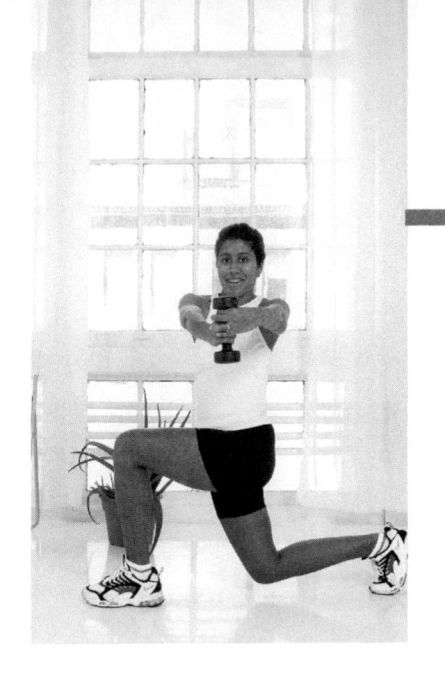

CONTENTS

PART ONE

You're a Mom!

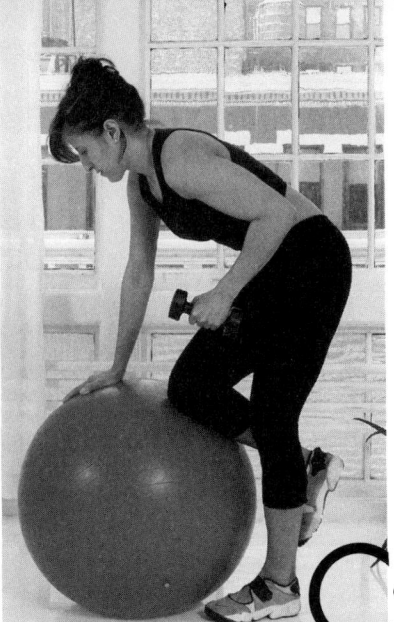

ongratulations! Your bundle of joy has arrived! My, how life has changed. No one knows better than you that pregnancy is an amazing journey. Not only has your body gone through a round of intense changes over the course of the last nine months, you are also experiencing another series of dramatic and emotional changes now that you've given birth. The impact on your body can leave you utterly exhausted! I've often heard from women that birthing a baby should qualify for an Olympic event. It can be compared with a long-distance, strength-training, and power event all at once. Pregnancy and childbirth place extreme stress on the body. Whether your baby's birth was at home or in the hospital, vaginal or cesarean, medicated or natural, your body has been through tremendous stress.

At the same time, you're experiencing the absolute joy of having a baby. The early days and weeks are packed with sweet moments with your little one. Unfortunately, your days may also include little sleep, your baby's needy siblings, a colicky baby, and work demands.

And let's not forget about physical discomfort. You may be feeling pain that you never thought was possible. With all of these things going on at the same time, most women find it a long road when it comes to getting back their pre-pregnancy bodies.

CHAPTER 1

Postpartum and Physical Changes

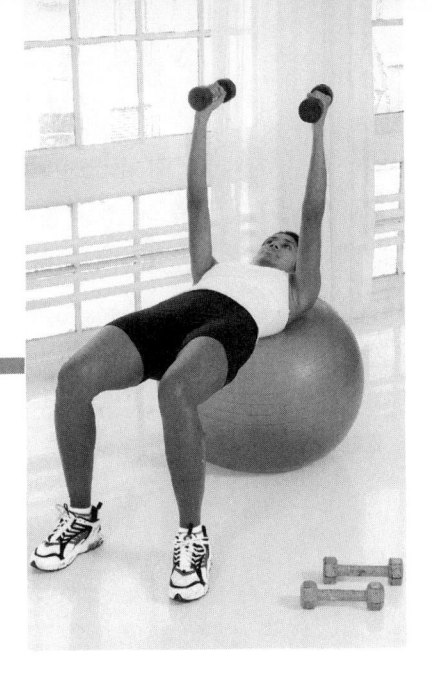

S ome of the most common physical changes that occur after having a baby make it especially difficult to start exercising. They are:

Bleeding

Lochia, or bloody vaginal discharge after birth, will start to disappear after several weeks. It is very common for the bleeding to stop and start intermittently during this time. Vaginal bleeding after a cesarean birth will usually be less than after a vaginal birth.

After-Birth Contractions

After giving birth, your uterus is still undergoing a series of changes in order to get back to its original size. The uterus shrinks from approximately the size of a basketball during pregnancy, to the size of a grapefruit after delivery, to the size of a pear six weeks postpartum. You will have a sensation similar to contractions, although not as painful. Breast-feeding may make these contractions worse, as the baby's sucking releases a hormone called oxytocin that contracts the uterus. These contractions should disappear after a couple of weeks. Lying on your stomach may help with the pain (unless you've had a C-section), as may keeping your bladder empty.

Breast Engorgement

When your milk supply comes in, two to four days after delivery, your breasts may become painful and firm. Fullness is a result of an increase in blood flow, which prepares your breasts for increased milk production. If you are not breast-feeding, the pain and swelling may subside within a few days. Snug-fitting bras may help; try to avoid getting warm water directly on your breasts, as this may increase milk production. If you are breast-feeding, frequent nursing will help keep your breasts soft. It may take a few days to get on a schedule with your baby to prevent engorgement. Using a breast pump to release a little breast milk may help, as may applying ice several times a day.

Pain When Urinating

Since the bladder and urethra are next to the bruised birth canal, difficulty urinating is common for new moms. If you were under anesthesia during a C-section, you may also have problems urinating. Drinking water immediately after delivery will help. Be sure to soak your bottom in warm water to promote healing.

Episiotomy

If you've had an episiotomy, good hygiene is essential during healing. Soaking in warm water three to four times a day will help soothe the soreness. Ice packs are recommended until the swelling is gone. A mild pain reliever or medication prescribed by your doctor will also help.

Perineum Pain

You may be sore and swollen in this area after birth. Keeping the perineum clean with soap and water will encourage healing.

Hemorrhoids

Hemorrhoids can develop due to the weight and the pressure of the baby, from the force of pushing during labor, and from constipation. Taking a hot bath three to four times a day, applying cold packs containing witch hazel, and sleeping on your side to take pressure off the veins of the rectum may help.

Fatigue

All new mothers experience some fatigue postpartum, whether they exercised throughout pregnancy or not. This may last for weeks, as your body tries to recover from the marathon that is pregnancy. Exercise will help (see suggestions in Part 2); however, recognize that your body has gone through a lot of changes. Give yourself time—and a break!

Physical Changes Due to Hormone Levels

After birth, your hormones continue to shift. These are common symptoms as your hormones stabilize:

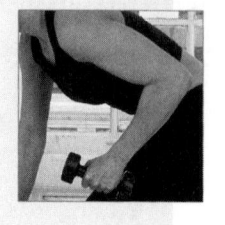

- **HOT FLASHES**
- **SWELLING**
- **DRY SKIN**
- **MOOD SWINGS**
- **INSOMNIA/NIGHT SWEATS**
- **HAIR LOSS (TEMPORARY)**

The American College of Obstetricians and Gynecologists reminds new moms that many of the physical changes that took place during pregnancy will persist four to six weeks after giving birth.

So, with all of these things going on at the same time, just how does a new mom begin to exercise? *Gradually!* During my career as a personal trainer, I've advised many women just how to get started during this crucial time. Getting rid of that "bundle of fat" may not be easy, nor may it be on your top-ten list. The first thing I say to my anxious clients is "Relax, don't worry, and get started!" Now is the time to investigate an exercise program to get back into pre-pregnancy form—not only for the moms who stayed fit and active during pregnancy, not only for the moms who are exercise beginners, but also for the moms who have children already and have not been able to lose the weight from their last pregnancy.

Now that you've had your baby, exercise and good nutrition are the keys to returning to your pre-pregnancy shape. The longer you wait to exercise after you've had your baby, the longer it will take to drop the extra weight gained during pregnancy. For those who remained active for the whole nine months, great! It will be that much easier to shed the weight. However, also know that you may not be able to pick up where you left off. Start slowly, and ease into an exercise routine. If you've just started exercising, good for you. However, keep it manageable and start slowly. Ten minutes a day may be enough in the beginning. Remember, as with any exercise program, consult your doctor before starting.

Good nutrition and eating habits are also imperative for shedding the excess pounds after having a baby. Breast-feeding and non-breast-feeding moms will have different nutritional needs; however, the term "dieting" should be removed from the vocabulary of *all* moms. This book will give nutritional tips and suggestions for moms, whether breast-feeding or not.

Recovery after pregnancy can take a long time. All bodies are different; some women can take longer than others to return to their pre-pregnancy shape. I tell all of my clients to give themselves a year to regain their bodies. Exercise should not be put on the back burner, however, as it is a crucial component in getting on the road to recovery. A balanced, safe, goal-oriented exercise program can help women get back their strength as well as tone and tighten muscles that were stretched during pregnancy. Generally, if you were active during pregnancy, you can resume a light workout a few days after your delivery. If you had a cesarean section, you will need more time to heal. If you're a newcomer to fitness, you'll need to start exercising more slowly.

Weight Gain/Loss After Pregnancy

The average weight gain during pregnancy is twenty-five to thirty-five pounds. During birth, moms lose about twelve to fifteen pounds, leaving about thirteen to twenty pounds of excess weight to lose in the postnatal period. This is when it gets tough. The last extra pounds can be hard to get rid of. However, there's good news: The consistent, safe exercise program described in this book can help you do that.

Research has indicated that women who begin to exercise right after (uncomplicated) delivery tend to lose more weight in the first six weeks than mothers who do not exercise then. Only about 35 percent of women exercise after giving birth. Studies indicate that if you worked out during pregnancy, you will tend to start exercising right after delivery.

Some women are concerned that exercise may impact their ability to breast-feed. No research supports that notion. Your body will tell you how active to be.

Not only do new moms have to deal with shedding excess weight gain, but also the physical demands of motherhood take a toll on the body. New moms have to deal with lifting and carrying their baby *and* heavy diaper bags, strollers, and car seats, which can leave them vulnerable to pain and injury. This book will suggest techniques for strengthening those affected muscle groups, such as the lower-back and abdominal areas. The core muscle groups are areas of the body that should not be overlooked after delivery. Strengthening them helps restore the body to optimal functioning and helps prepare women for the many physical demands of motherhood.

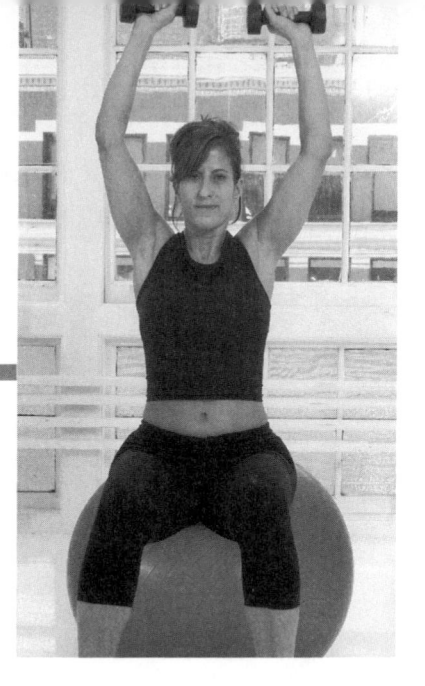

CHAPTER 2

Frequently Asked Questions

Throughout the years, I have discovered a pattern to the concerns and questions new moms have about exercise. Most women are reluctant to start exercise programs right after having a baby. Here are the top-ten frequently asked questions of the postpartum mom:

   1. QUESTION: How long will it take for me to get back to my prepregnancy figure?

   ANSWER: First, after you've given birth, accept the fact that you will have gained an extra few pounds. But then just take one look at your sleeping baby and you will be reminded that gaining and losing the weight is worth it. Generally, it takes up to six months to a year to lose the excess weight. We all know of women who have bounced back after two weeks. They appear just as fit as they were before pregnancy. This is not the norm. Your goal should be to lose two to four pounds a month. You may lose less if you are breast-feeding.

2. QUESTION: I've heard that losing weight while nursing is not recommended. Is this true?

ANSWER: Losing more than four pounds a week is not encouraged while you're breast-feeding. The body stores toxins in fat, and if you lose weight too quickly, there is a possibility that the toxins will enter your breast milk. Also, burning a large number of calories in a short period of time may affect your milk production. Gradual weight loss, combined with exercise, is the recommended course of action.

3. QUESTION: Is it safe to exercise with weights after having a baby?

ANSWER: Strength training (using weights or your own body weight) is an excellent way to tone muscle groups that were weakened during pregnancy and labor. Later in the book I will discuss the benefits of core strength training, or strengthening of the abdominal muscles and lower back.

4. QUESTION: When can I start exercising after I've had my baby?

ANSWER: Good news! Years ago, exercise during pregnancy was discouraged and not recommended until six months after birth. Times have changed. The American College of Obstetricians and Gynecologists recently reversed those recommendations and now say it's okay to start exercising right away, as long as you feel up to it and get the approval of your doctor. Exercise actually promotes healing. If you've had a cesarean section, you will have to wait a bit longer to start your exercise program, as your incision will need to heal. If you were lucky enough to exercise right up to giving birth and had a normal vaginal delivery, you can probably start light exercise days afterward.

5. QUESTION: How do I know if I'm exercising too soon or too much?

ANSWER: Women experience a bloody vaginal discharge called lochia during the first few weeks after delivery. This is normal; however, if the flow becomes redder and heavier, this may be a sign that you're trying to do too much, too soon. Stop exercising and notify your doctor.

It is important to listen to your body. If you're finding yourself extremely fatigued, it may be too soon for exercise, or you may be working out too hard.

6. QUESTION: Is biking safe during my postpartum recovery?

ANSWER: That really depends on the type of delivery you had. If you had some tissue damage during delivery or stitches from an episiotomy (an incision made to enlarge the vaginal opening) or to repair tearing of the vagina, you may need more time to heal. Biking is not recommended immediately following a C-section; you will have to let your incision heal before including it in your exercise plan. Doughnut seats are recommended to relieve pressure if you find yourself sensitive when riding a bike.

7. QUESTION: What is the best way for me to lose weight postpartum?

ANSWER: Practicing good eating habits and getting a balanced workout, one that includes cardiovascular exercise and strength training, with obtainable goals, are the best ways to lose weight safely and effectively. Walking, swimming, biking, and jogging (when your doctor says it's okay) are great forms of aerobic exercise. Light resistance training will help build strength and restore tone.

Listen to your body; it will tell you when to lengthen your workouts. In the beginning, the luxurious forty-five-minute workout may have to remain a distant memory.

8. QUESTION: Are genetics a factor when trying to get back into pre-pregnancy shape?

ANSWER: Yes! How easily you get your old body back depends on many things, such as genetics, how much you exercised during pregnancy, and whether you had complications during pregnancy and delivery. Everyone has a certain body type, and you should work with what you have. Don't compare yourself with pictures in a magazine or with your friends. It took nine months to have your baby; give yourself that much time to get back into shape.

9. QUESTION: Does it matter if I work out before I breast-feed?

ANSWER: Always try to exercise *after* nursing your baby so your breasts won't feel uncomfortable and full. Try to avoid exercises that make your breasts sore and tender.

10. QUESTION: How do I get rid of stretch marks?

ANSWER: Stretch marks are a result of rapid weight gain and are common during pregnancy. This stretching of the skin results in red or purple lines across the lower stomach, thighs, or breasts during pregnancy. Stretch marks are permanent, but they become less noticeable once the weight is lost and the skin shrinks back to normal. Usually the tendency to get stretch marks is hereditary, and some women have the misfortune of getting more than others. Even though stretch marks are inevitable for some, keeping the skin moist and eating well are some of the best ways to prevent them and help make them less noticeable.

You may be asking yourself, "Does the *Buff Moms* workout guide really work?" Yes, it does, and I have a couple of success stories of its exercises and those from *Buff Moms-to-Be* to prove it. Sure, at times these women found it hard to get motivated and find the time to fit exercise in, but once they got going, they felt better and started to see the results of their hard work. This is even true for women who hadn't lost the weight they'd gained from previous pregnancies! Here's Jennifer's story. . . .

It wasn't until she gave birth to her second child that Jennifer's weight problem began. At five-four, she weighed 145 pounds postpartum, and she hadn't lost the weight from her previous pregnancy. "I was always skinny and never worried about my weight," Jennifer says. Not only did the demands of her two small children take up her time, but she was also working full-time as vice president of an investment firm. When her weight jumped to 150 pounds nine months after having her baby, she knew that she needed to do something. "I looked in the mirror, looked at old photos, and still appeared pregnant! I couldn't believe that my weight had gotten to that point," she says.

After checking with her doctor, Jennifer started to walk two to three times a week and followed the exercise suggestions in *Buff Moms*. "It didn't matter that I wasn't exactly a 'new' mom. This plan got me going and guided me back to a healthier way of life."

Jennifer found the time to work out by asking her husband, family, and friends to babysit so she could exercise at least three times a week. She also looked at her eating habits and started to make better nutritional choices. "It was amazing how much I was eating. I would taste the kids' food to make sure it was okay, have my dinner, then finish what the children didn't eat!"

As she implemented these changes, Jennifer started to lose one to one and a half pounds a week. "I was so excited; I was on my way to becoming a Buff Mom. The ironic part about all this was that I was able to keep up my workout commitment because I felt healthier with all the new energy I had." Over the next six months, Jennifer lost ten pounds. "I feel great; this plan certainly helped me get started and focused. My kids see me exercising, and I know I'm teaching them valuable habits."

Virginia has brought three magnificent children into this world in the last three years. She has watched her body go from 135 pounds to 165 pounds then back down to 135 pounds three times. During each pregnancy, she worked really hard at staying in shape while eating plenty of the right kinds of food to help her baby grow to a healthy size.

"To eat healthy and stay in shape is a lot easier said than done, especially when people are saying, 'Oh, have more, you're eating for two!' Basically, it comes down to eating right, sleeping, and exercising. I am a firm believer that a woman's body that is actually reproducing another human being is like the most complex computer and needs at least eight hours of sleep to run successfully. I also believe that regular exercise is key to having more energy and making my deliveries easier. Following the *Buff Moms-to-Be* exercises has made it easier for me to incorporate exercise into my daily life. I don't have the time to figure out my own exercise program."

Virginia found that breaking the stereotypes and jokes about pregnant women was hard. "We are surrounded by pictures of pregnant women eating ice cream and two pieces of chocolate cake. Eating for two is encouraged! I really had to buckle down and remember that I must eat the foods that contain nutritional value for me and my growing baby. I feel that really taking care of my body and myself by eating right and exercising when I carried my children has prepared me a great deal for being a healthy mom. Putting the baby's health as first priority is the first of many sacrifices a mother will make for her child. Creating a child is truly a miracle!

"I really owe my three physically challenging yet successful quick labors to exercising through my pregnancies. I feel that delivering a baby is like being in a marathon, yet you have not been told the date, time, and place. In that case, you must eat right, have had adequate sleep, and be in shape when it's time. I never pushed my pregnant body; I just felt that it was important to incorporate exercise into my daily life three times a week. Getting in shape after I had my babies was also easier. I have tested the exercise-while-pregnant theory three times and now that my youngest is four months old, I can say the *Buff Moms-to-Be* program worked every time! I am now back to my original size. I was able to start exercising right away after giving birth, thanks to staying active and fit throughout my pregnancy. I continue to exercise daily; soon my three little ones will be joining their mommy!"

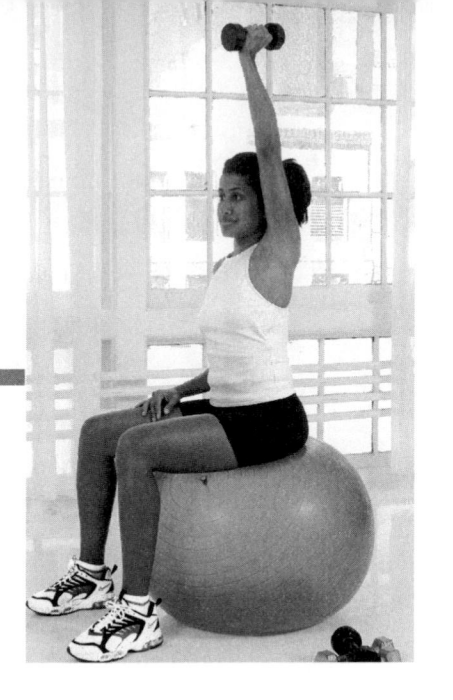

CHAPTER 3

Buff Nutrition

Exercise is certainly one of the main components of getting back to your old shape; however, a good nutritional plan is another vital piece of the puzzle. Whether you breast-feed or formula-feed your newborn, making good food choices and exercising are your best bets in reaching your goals.

Within a few days of having your baby, you may lose two to four pounds of fluid, two pounds from the shrinking uterus, and several pounds from the delivery of the baby and amniotic fluid. Of course, you'll still weigh more after the baby is born than you did before you were pregnant. Usually, the remaining weight is stored as fat. Getting rid of the excess weight won't happen overnight.

Watching your calories is crucial; however, a breast-feeding mom has different requirements than a non-breast-feeding mother. Usually, a non-breast-feeding mom needs a caloric intake of 1,500 to 2,000 calories a day (average), whereas if you are breast-feeding, you may need 2,000 to 2,300 calories a day. Also, both breast-feeding moms and non-breast-feeding moms need to get plenty of calcium and protein in their diet.

Many new moms feel zapped of energy. Having a baby is a wonderful experience, but it can be an exhausting one as well. Try cutting back on caffeine, and make sure your meals are stocked with protein. Protein is what sustains energy. Also, try to eat often. Usually, eating every three to four hours will maintain good energy.

Sleep can be a dilemma for many new moms (and not-so-new moms!). Research proves that new moms get only four to six hours of sleep a night. Getting sleep is important, especially when you start to exercise. Try taking naps with your baby, or ask family for help.

Nutrition for the Non-nursing Mom

If you are a non-nursing mom, losing weight may be a priority, but doing it sensibly and in a healthy way is vital to keeping up your energy levels and staying a step ahead of the demands of your baby.

You should eat nutritious foods and have in mind the goal of cutting back 250 to 300 calories a day. Slow weight loss will help you shed weight that stays off. Your goal should be to lose no more than one to one and a half pounds a week. Keep in mind that in order to do this, you must burn more calories than you take in. This is where exercise comes in.

Your exercise plan (discussed in Part Two) should be a program that incorporates small, obtainable goals. Try to get the most nutrition from each calorie; be smart in your food choices. The key is *not* to go on a diet, especially for the first three months after having your baby. Instead, focus on healthy eating. The two biggest mistakes a new mom can make are to go on a crash diet and to continue eating junk food. The American Medical Association suggests that a diet should be "nutritionally sound." This is a diet low in fat (not fat-free) and nutrient-dense (full of vitamins and minerals) and high in fiber. Whether or not your goal is to lose weight, these recommendations apply to all. Educate yourself and find out what the foods you are eating contain.

Buff Nutritional Tips for the Non-nursing Mom*

1. The majority of the calories you eat should come from carbohydrates and whole grains. Eat six to eleven servings a day of whole-grain cereals, breads, pasta, or rice.

2. You should strive for three to five servings of vegetables and two to four servings of fruit a day.

3. Two to three servings of low-fat milk, yogurt, or cheeses are recommended per day.

4. To balance your diet, eat two to three servings of lean meat, fish, poultry (skinless), or eggs a day.

5. Eat regularly and often. This means eating small meals throughout the day. One tends to overeat when cutting back to one or two meals per day.

6. It's okay to snack! Just think before you do. Make better choices about your foods and have healthy snacks available when you feel a craving coming on.

7. Write down what you eat. This is a great way to look back at the end of the day and see when/where you had a weak moment. It will also help you see if you're getting the recommended food servings I discussed earlier.

*Butters, oils, and fats should be used in small amounts. Use your good judgment.

8. Clean up and throw away! You may find that when you are cooking for the whole family, you're finishing meals for them. These are calories that add up at the end of the day.

9. Make time for yourself to sit down and eat. Just because you have a busy schedule doesn't mean you have to sacrifice good eating practices. Eating in a rush only welcomes unhealthy choices.

10. Drink eight to twelve glasses of water a day.

Nutrition for the Nursing Mom

Breast-feeding may help with weight loss during the twelve months after giving birth. During pregnancy, your body acquires fat deposits in many different places. Breast-feeding uses these fat deposits to produce milk. Nursing can burn over five hundred calories per day. However, you should not rely on this for losing weight. A sensible nutritional plan combined with exercise will help you achieve your weight-loss goals. By eating healthfully, you will not only speed up your recovery, but your baby will enjoy all the nutrients and minerals that are needed for strong growth and health.

If you gained no more than twenty-two to thirty pounds, and you're breast-feeding, the number of calories you consume should not fall below 1,800 per day. Remember, you're still eating for two: everything you eat directly affects the health of your new baby. Plus, by choosing healthful food, you will have more energy and strength to get you through the day and help you regain your prebaby figure.

Buff Nutritional Tips for the Nursing Mom

1. Try to have at least five servings of fresh fruits and vegetables a day. Include at least one serving of a dark orange vegetable, two

servings of a dark green leafy vegetable, and one serving of a citrus fruit. This will assure that you and your baby are getting the necessary minerals and vitamins each day.

2. Increase your calcium intake. Try to drink three glasses of low-fat or fat-free milk each day. It has been recommended that 1,000 milligrams of calcium should be consumed daily. Other foods rich in calcium are calcium-fortified orange juice and soy milk, and low-fat cheeses and yogurt.

3. Eat lots of whole grains. Your daily menu should include six servings of whole-grain foods.

4. Pep and protein! Include two to three servings of fish, poultry (skinless), lean or extra-lean meats, or dried beans a day.

5. Water, water, water! Drink eight to twelve glasses each day. Caffeine is okay in moderation. Limit your alcohol consumption to eight ounces of wine or two beers a day.

6. Balance your calories. When you're nursing, your body requires more vitamins and minerals for you and your baby. Choose foods that are high in nutrients to ensure optimum health for the two of you.

7. Ask your doctor if you should take vitamin supplements while nursing.

Bottom line, this is *not* the time to go on a fad or crash diet. A diet with too few calories may reduce your milk supply. Keep track of what you're eating—a food diary is great for the nursing mom as well. Starving is never the answer to losing weight; instead, eat small, healthful meals consistently throughout the day.

Both nursing and non-nursing moms should remember a few basic tips when trying to cut out extra, nonessential calories:

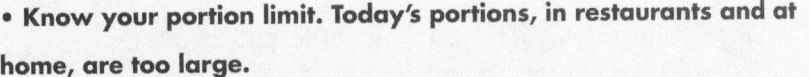

- **Know your portion limit. Today's portions, in restaurants and at home, are too large.**
- **Watch in-between-meal snacks. Instead of dips, chips, cheeses, and pizza, try veggies, fruit, and low-fat options.**
- **The skin on meats and poultry contains a lot of unnecessary calories. Choose lean meats and poultry without the skin.**
- **Drink water with your meals. It fills you up, so you're less likely to overeat.**
- **Watch your consumption of juices and sodas. They contain a lot of sugar, and less sugar equals fewer calories.**

Most of all, be patient, be realistic, and set obtainable goals.

It is important for new moms to realize that their nutrient levels were depleted during pregnancy. Replenishing these nutrients during postpartum recovery is crucial. If you are breast-feeding, the nutrient depletion may be more than for the non-breast-feeding mom. Women who have lost a great deal of blood during pregnancy or had a cesarean section may have a greater depletion of nutrients. Some common signs of nutritional depletion:

- **FATIGUE**
- **INSOMNIA**
- **LONELINESS**
- **SADNESS**
- **PROBLEMS DIGESTING CERTAIN FOODS**
- **IRRITABILITY, MOODINESS**
- **LACK OF ENERGY**

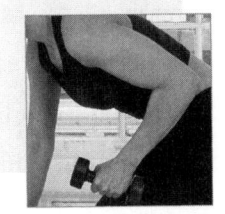

It is vital for women to recognize these common signs. It is also crucial for new moms to incorporate a healthful diet, exercise program, and, if needed, nutritional supplements into their daily life.

The Veteran Mom

Many women trying to lose weight are veteran moms, women who still have pounds to lose from previous pregnancies. Often, they find themselves too busy to exercise. Well, there's good news: It is possible to use this guide and get back into shape even if you've been a mom for a year or more.

The exercises described in Part Two and the nutritional guidelines I described earlier will get you on your way. If you feel overwhelmed by starting a fitness program and maintaining a healthful diet, don't worry; it's crucial that you keep things simple and manageable. You live a busy life; trying to balance all of these things can leave the veteran mom exhausted!

As you get started with an exercise program, look at your eating habits. You may discover, after a year or more, that you're still eating for two. You look in the mirror and see that you never lost your postpartum weight. You may even have forgotten what your pre-pregnancy body looked like.

Well, just remember to take it slow and don't expect to lose the weight in a few weeks. Your weight depends a lot on genetics and body type, so don't get fixated on a number. To estimate your ideal weight (within a 10 percent variation), figure one hundred pounds for five feet in height and add five pounds for each inch over five feet tall. For example, if you are five feet, four inches tall, your ideal weight will be somewhere between 110 and 130 pounds.

Remember, gradual weight loss should be your focus, not losing large amounts of weight quickly. Consider losing one to one and a half pounds a week as excellent progress.

Cutting Calories

Basically, to lose one pound a week, you should cut five hundred calories from your diet each day. To estimate how many calories you can consume daily and still lose weight, multiply your current weight by thirteen if your activity level is moderate.* The result is the number of calories you need to maintain your current weight.

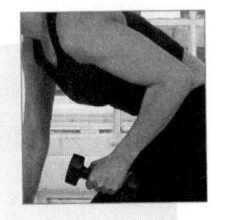

For example, a mom who does moderate exercise and weighs 145 pounds:

$$145 \times 13 = 1{,}885 \text{ cal/day}$$
$$- 500 \text{ cal.}$$
$$= 1{,}385 \text{ cal/day}$$

Women also need to know that their daily caloric intake must not fall below 1,200 calories per day, which their bodies need to function healthfully. And remember, if you are breast-feeding, you need an additional five hundred to seven hundred calories per day for your nursing baby. Brand-new moms should not eat fewer than 1,500 calories per day, in order to stay strong and energetic for their new baby.

*This formula only works if you are doing some form of moderate exercise. It is not recommended that you rely solely on cutting calories to lose weight.

A realistic goal to shoot for: your body weight in the year before your last pregnancy or, if it has been more than five years since you were pregnant, your best weight in those five years (to account for the age factor and metabolic slowdown, see pages 84–85). Think back and get an accurate idea of what you really looked like, since that will be an ideal that is achievable.

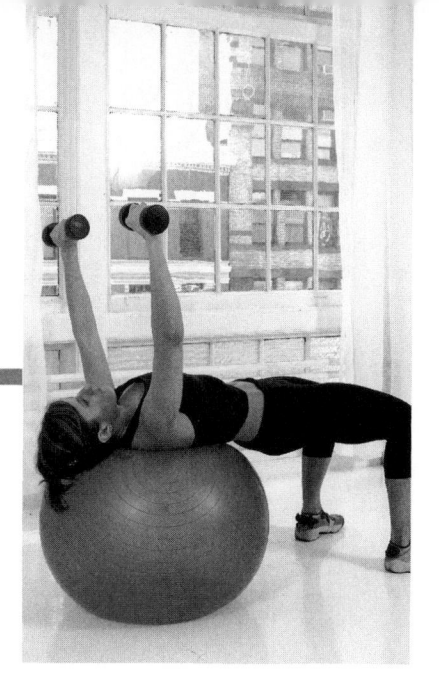

CHAPTER 4

Fitting Exercise In

All mothers, veteran and new, may find it impossible to exercise. I tell my clients over and over, don't be shy, and ask for help. That is the only way you'll find the time, especially with everything else you have to do. Instead of thinking two hours in the gym, think short bursts of exercise two or three times a day. If your kids are old enough, bring them along on bike rides or put them in a baby stroller or jogger. Don't make exercise last on the to-do list. Most new moms are overwhelmed by the new responsibility of caring for their newborn. The first few weeks after delivery are filled with learning how to do baby things for the first time. However, finding a few minutes a day to exercise will not only help you lose weight but will help release stress, allow you to relax, and speed up your recovery time. The key is to find ways to fit activities you enjoy into your daily lifestyle. Here are a few tips for fitting fitness in:

- **Ask for help!** Yes, don't be afraid to hand off your baby to your husband, partner, mom, dad, or friends for an hour. Use this time to rejuvenate and heal.

- **Ask friends to make dinner.** Having a prepared meal or two on hand can save some time in the kitchen and leave some time for the workout.

- **Hire a housecleaner,** one of the best luxuries a new mom can have. Use that time to sneak in a workout.

- **Bring the baby along.** Whether you use a gym or work out at home or with a videotape, bring the baby along. Most gyms offer a babysitting service while you work out. Buff Moms can be used in the gym as well.

- **Exercise while the baby is napping.** Make sure he isn't close enough for you to disturb his sleep, but close enough so you'll hear him when he wakes. Or, invest in a baby monitor.

- **Exercise with your baby.** Take your baby for a walk in a stroller or front-carrier. When your baby is old enough and has developed more strength and better head control, you'll be able to place him in a bike trailer or jogging stroller. See pages 111–114 for exercises you can do with your baby.

- **Investigate exercise videos** that you can do with your baby. These can be quite active and fun as you keep your baby in a front-carrier.

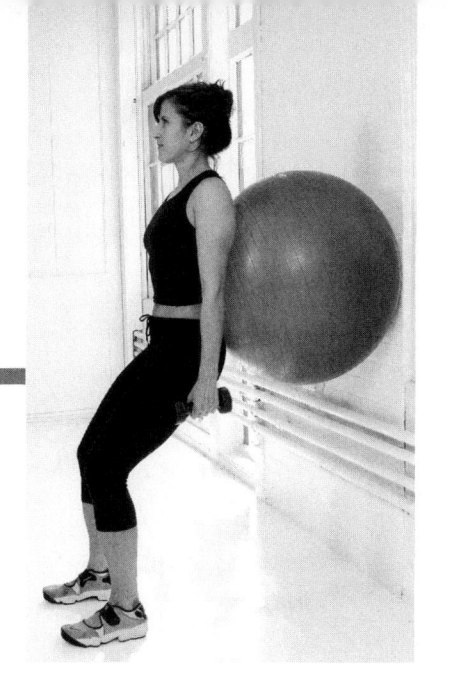

CHAPTER 5

The Baby Blues

Many new moms suffer from the blues right after having a baby. Research has shown that 50 to 75 percent of recent moms will experience some form of the baby blues. This shouldn't be surprising, considering all of the new demands being made on them. Many moms also experience doubt about their ability to care for a baby. Exhaustion is also prevalent. Your baby requires a lot of time, and you and your partner may not be used to this in the beginning. You may experience episodes of unexplained crying, mood swings, lack of appetite, and the general feeling of having lost your sense of self. Such feelings are normal and usually go away after a week or two.

Postpartum Depression

Postpartum depression and psychosis are more severe and devastating than baby blues. PPD has been recognized since ancient times. In 700 B.C., Hippocrates described the emotional problems associated with childbearing. Unfortunately, the medical community has for many years failed to acknowledge and formally recognize the existence of a depressive disorder related directly to childbearing. Even today, controversy exists about how to define and classify the depression that occurs during the postpartum period. The American College of Obstetricians and Gynecologists estimates that one out of ten new mothers experiences postpartum depression. If any of the feelings listed below last longer than two to four weeks after the birth of your baby, share them with your doctor, partner, family, and friends. You may be experiencing symptoms of postpartum depression, which is treatable.

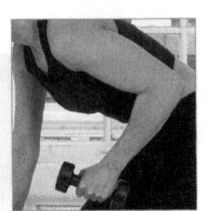

Common symptoms of postpartum depression include:

ANXIETY

INSOMNIA

PANIC

DIFFICULTY CONCENTRATING

CRYING

LETHARGY

FEELINGS OF GUILT

LOW SELF-ESTEEM

DECREASED APPETITE

MOOD SWINGS

FEELINGS OF HOPELESSNESS

IRRITABILITY

FEELING OVERWHELMED

Current research has not determined the exact cause of PPD. What is known is that pregnancy can wreak havoc on the hormones. The hormonal changes that you experience after having a baby can be quite dramatic. Estrogen and progesterone levels increase during pregnancy then decrease dramatically after delivery. Research has indicated a link between PPD and rapidly declining hormone levels. Changes in blood levels of certain steroids, cortisol, and aldosterone have also been linked to PPD.

The enormous stress of caring for a newborn also can create mood changes for new mothers. The physical exhaustion, sleep deprivation, and social isolation that follow childbirth all can contribute to the depth of depression moms may have after delivery.

Research also indicates that half of women who become depressed after one delivery will experience PPD after future deliveries. If you have a history of depression, this should be discussed with your doctor during and after pregnancy.

Exercise is a great way to boost endorphins, which in turn can improve one's mood. Although the motivation to exercise may not be there, it is important to make attempts at exercising, even if only for ten or fifteen minutes a day.

Remember, don't be too hard on yourself: adjusting to motherhood is one of the hardest challenges in life. Having a new little addition to your life is a twenty-four-hour-a-day job. Once you get used to your new life, these challenges will get easier. And if you're good to yourself, these anxious feelings should subside after a few weeks. Enjoy your baby and this wonderful change in your life.

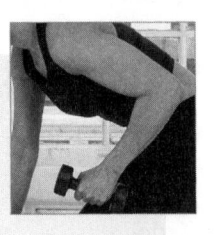

Again, talking to your partner and friends, as well as your doctor, can help. Here are some other tips:

- Exercising even ten minutes here and there will help tremendously.
- Get plenty of rest. It sounds impossible, but enlist the help of your partner. Don't overload yourself with tasks that are unimportant.
- Get as much information on motherhood as you can before you have your baby.
- Try to eat foods that are rich in nutrients.
- Stay away from dieting.
- Drink plenty of fluids.
- Take some time for yourself—away from the baby!
- Walk around the block.
- Ask for help with the housework.
- Seek support groups—investigate your church, local clinic, or health center.
- Find other new moms.
- Treat yourself!
- Enjoy every day and your new wonderful, beautiful baby.

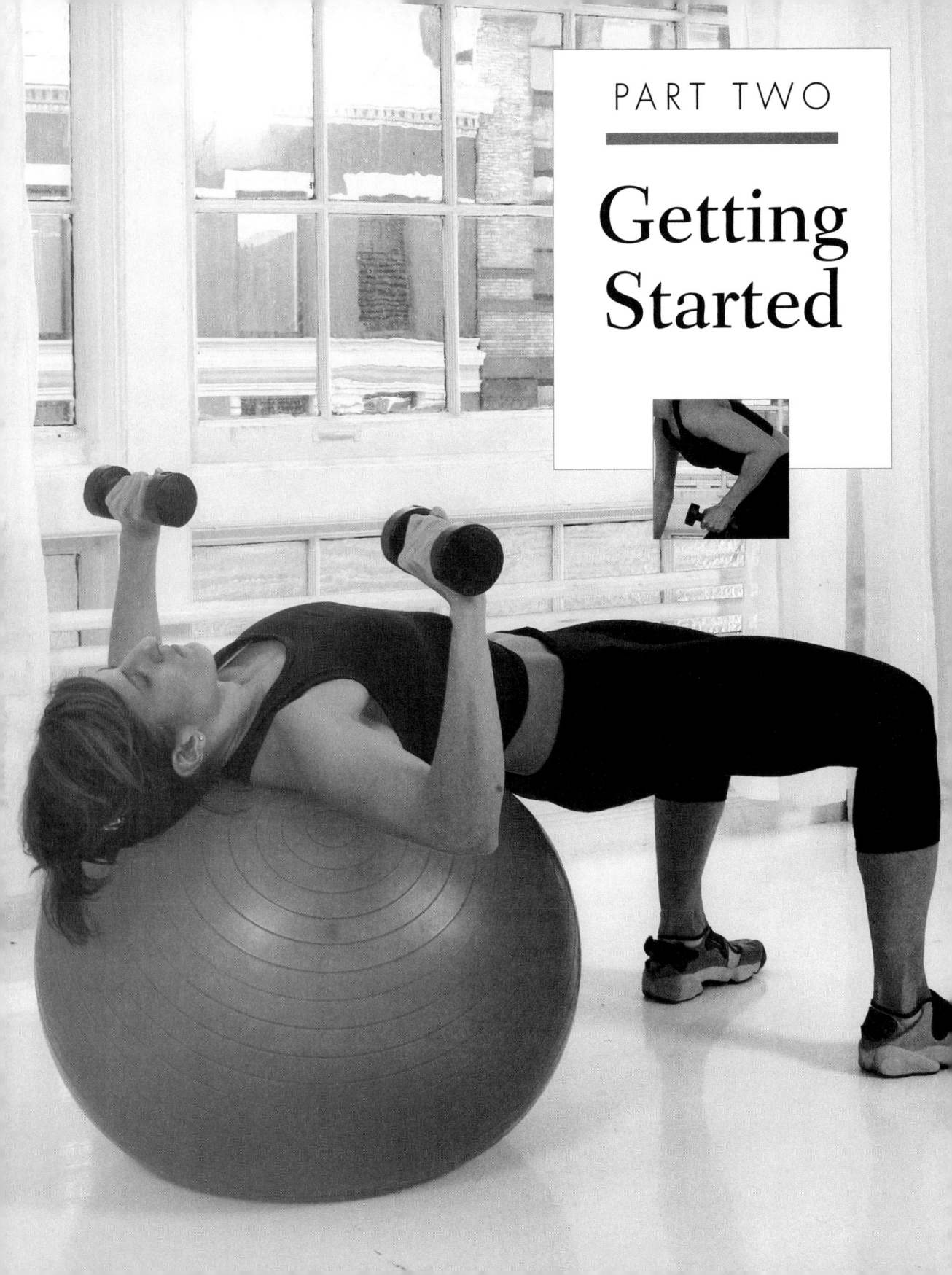

PART TWO

Getting Started

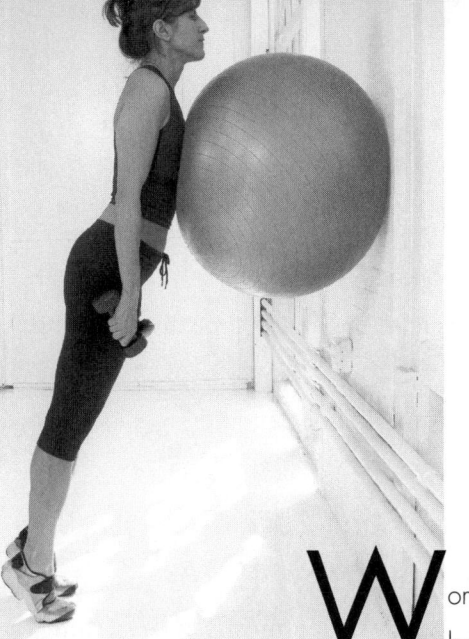

Women who exercised regularly during pregnancy may not be capable of their usual workout postpartum. Weight gain and the decline in activity associated with pregnancy contribute to decreased fitness. Ligament laxity associated with increased levels of relaxin during pregnancy may increase a woman's risk of injury from postpartum exercise. Although relaxin levels return to normal within the first week after delivery, laxity may persist for three months after delivery.

Exercise has to be a priority, part of your daily routine. Yes, it takes commitment. It also takes planning, compromise, and loads of flexibility. Keep in mind that staying fit over the long haul is more important than getting into shape right after giving birth. So choose the fitness level appropriate for you. Physical fitness is essential to good health. You owe it to yourself and you owe it to your family.

Benefits of Mom-and-Baby Exercise After Childbirth

Benefits for Mom:

    Enhances psychological well-being

    Assists with regaining of muscle strength and tone after childbirth

    Reduces back discomfort

    Provides a naturally progressive workout—mothers get more fit as babies gain weight

Benefits for Baby:

    Promotes bonding with Mom

    Stimulation—babies enjoy the movement, music, and watching the video's smiling moms and babies

Cardiovascular Exercise

With any exercise program, cardiovascular exercise is one of the most important components of fitness. Cardiovascular fitness is the ability of your lungs, heart, and vascular system to efficiently transport oxygen to your muscles. Aerobic exercise strengthens cardiovascular fitness. *Aerobic* means "with, or in the presence of, oxygen." Walking, jogging, and biking are all examples of aerobic exercises—exercises that utilize oxygen. Incorporating aerobic exercise into your life will improve your cardiovascular fitness because your body learns to utilize its oxygen supply more efficiently. When you utilize oxygen more efficiently, your heart doesn't have to work as hard to pump blood and oxygen throughout your body. This results in a stronger, more efficient heart. Cardiovascular exercise is crucial for maintaining and losing weight. During aerobic exercise, your body expends a lot of energy because you process and utilize more oxygen. This energy is measured in calories. For every liter of oxygen (or one kilogram of body weight) used during an aerobic activity, the

BUFF EXERCISE POINTERS

- **Start by consulting your doctor. Once you get his okay, listen to your body. Moms who had a C-section may need additional time to heal.**

- **Resume exercise gradually. Some of the physical changes that took place during pregnancy may persist four to six weeks after delivery. Moderation is the key; progress slowly.**

- **Develop an exercise plan. Think it through before you start.**

- **If you develop severe or chronic pain, vaginal bleeding, faintness, generalized edema, palpitations, nausea, shortness of breath, extreme fatigue, or muscle weakness, stop immediately and contact your doctor.**

- **Invest in a good pair of sneakers. Your feet may still be swollen following pregnancy.**

- **Nursing moms may need extra bra support. Make sure your bra fits snugly, whether you're nursing or not.**

- **Drink lots of fluids, preferably water.**

- **Balance your workouts with stretching, cardiovascular work, and strength training. Make sure to warm up and cool down properly.**

- **Make exercise a commitment. You're less likely to see results working out one day a week rather than three or four days a week.**

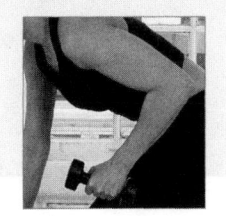

body spends five calories. The more energy you spend and the longer you exercise, the more oxygen is used and the more calories you will burn.

The key is to mix things up and find a form of exercise you like. In the beginning, walking will probably be the only cardiovascular exercise you can do. Slow walks during this initial period will not only help you feel you're getting back into a fitness routine, but will also help you relieve tension and get some fresh air. Don't push yourself—work to establish a regular routine and keep a steady pace. A full-fledged return to aerobic activities you participated in pre-pregnancy (or establishing a routine if you're a beginner) usually comes around the four-to-six-week-postpartum period. As you begin to feel better and you start to heal, gradually increase your cardio program and integrate the strength-training exercises that I outline, which target many of the major muscle groups. Other forms of cardiovascular activities include:

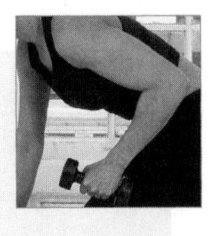

• **JOGGING** **Invest in a good pair of running shoes. In the beginning, start with walking. Once you feel stronger (about two to three weeks postpartum), alternate walking with jogging. For example, for every three minutes of walking, alternate with one minute of jogging.**

• **SWIMMING***

• **BIKING*** **A stationary bike can be a relatively economical piece of home-exercise equipment. (Stationary bikes can cost anywhere from a few hundred to thousands of dollars.) One downside is that it only works your lower body. If you have lower back pain, recumbent bikes may be better for you. However, they are a bit easier to use than upright bikes, and you may have to push yourself harder to stay in your target heart rate zone and achieve a beneficial workout. One thing to remember about stationary bikes is that if they will be placed near the baby, consider models equipped with a chain guard and a solid front wheel that covers the spokes to protect crawling children's fingers. Also, invest in a comfortable seat; it makes a world of difference.**

• **AEROBICS CLASSES** **low-impact in the beginning**

• **YOGA**

* Swimming and biking are excellent postpartum activities because they are non-weight-bearing aerobic exercises that can restore your cardiovascular conditioning without stressing the joints. However, if you had some tissue damage during delivery or had an episiotomy, you may need more time to heal before starting these activities.

For those not ready to do more than walk, yoga-based exercise is a great way to help your body and mind get back into shape after having your baby. With practice, positions and movements soon become second nature, enabling you to pick and choose the ones that feel most comfortable. Some of the yoga positions can be done as you are watching TV.

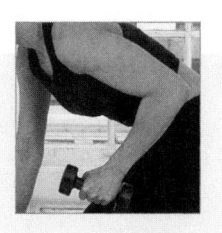

THE PHYSICAL BENEFITS OF YOGA:

• Better circulation of blood and lymph fluids

• Better breathing

• Improved muscle tone

• Greater strength and more flexibility

• Less tension and stiffness in your muscles and joints

• Relief from minor ailments or aches and pains (especially back pain)

• Improved energy levels and less fatigue

• Better posture

• A positive mental attitude

SCIENTIFIC STUDY HAS SHOWN THAT YOGA:

• Increases suppleness

• Improves cardiovascular efficiency and overall fitness though it does not involve vigorous exercise

• Lowers blood pressure

• Balances blood composition

Exercises to Avoid

There are some exercises that should be avoided the first few weeks after having your baby. Ballistic movements (bouncing) and deep flexion or extension of joints should be avoided because of the joint tissue laxity that continues after pregnancy. Jumping, activities that require quick changes of direction, and any type of jarring motion should be avoided to prevent possible stretching and dislocation of these joints. The knee, hip, and back are especially susceptible to injury during the first few weeks after pregnancy. Avoid exercising on hard surfaces such as pavement. Instead, use carpeted surfaces, grass, or padded mats.

Try to keep a consistent exercise schedule and give yourself plenty of warm-up, stretching, and cool-down time. Although stretching should be done cautiously because of joint laxity, it still should be done every day to regain flexibility.

Avoid exercising in the heat. Hydration is key during this transitional phase of resuming activity. Make your drink choice water, and try to stay away from fruit juices, as they tend to have a lot of sugar.

Monitoring Your Heart Rate

It is important that you monitor your heart rate as you begin to exercise postpartum. This also holds true for veteran moms just starting a fitness program. Consult your doctor on what your target heart rate should be and make sure you don't exceed it. A heart rate monitor may not be a bad investment to ensure you're not working out too hard. Heart rate monitors are worn on the body while exercising and let you know how many times your heart is beating per minute. You can also check your heart rate manually. Periodically during your workout, place your index and middle fingers in the groove on the side of your throat. Starting at zero, count how many times your heart beats in six seconds (a clock will help). Add a zero to that number. This is how many times approximately your heart is beating per minute.

Keeping track of your heart rate not only ensures that you're not working out too strenuously, but will help you determine if your cardiovascular fitness is improving.

Determining Your Target Heart Rate:

Your target heart rate range is the recommended heart rate range for safe and effective participation in aerobic activities. Calculating your

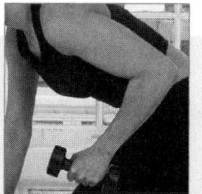

TARGET HEART RATE FORMULA*

                        220

Subtract your age   –

= your Maximum Heart Rate

Subtract your RHR from MHR   –

= your Heart Rate Reserve

Multiply your HRR by: x   .60   and   x   .80

                             =   =

Add your RHR to answers above +   +

= your Target Heart Rate   =   =

Example: a 30-year-old woman with an RHR of 70 BPM

220 – 30 = 190 (Maximum Heart Rate)

190 – 70 = 120 (Heart Rate Reserve)

120 x .60 = 72 and 120 x .80 = 96

72 + 70 = 142 and 96 + 70 = 166 (Target Heart Rate = 142 to 166 BPM)

* Remember, a doctor may recommend staying in the lower range of the target heart rate for the postpartum mom and the newcomer to fitness.

target rate requires you to know your resting heart rate (RHR) and to be able to locate and take an accurate pulse check during aerobic activities. Once you've calculated your RHR (count the number of beats you feel on your wrist or neck for six seconds, starting at zero, and then multiply that number by ten), you can determine your target heart rate zone.

Creating Your Home Gym

Getting back into your prebaby shape doesn't have to mean expensive gym memberships. An affordable, simple gym in your own home can make it much easier to keep your new fitness commitments. A home gym really comes in handy when it's not possible to go for a fitness walk or to an exercise class with your baby. A few good pieces of equipment will put you on your way to being a Buff Mom.

The equipment I suggest should cost you no more than sixty dollars. However, if you have the space and the extra money, a good machine set up in a convenient spot in your home may inspire you to work out whenever you have some free time. The cost is often no more than that of a one-year gym membership. The basic machines are treadmills, elliptical trainers, stair-steppers, and stationary bikes. However, if you don't want to invest in machines, you can still achieve your fitness goals with some other basic equipment.

Make sure your baby is in a secure infant seat, high chair, or playpen before beginning your workout. Since you'll be exercising indoors, try to use a fan or open a window to keep you comfortable.

You will be able to find all of the following items at your local sporting goods retailer.

Fitness Ball

Tired of doing basic crunches? Then get yourself a fitness ball. This over-size ball, once used for physical rehabilitation, is a staple in every gym. You can do hundreds of core-strengthening exercises with this versatile piece of gear. Strengthening the core muscle groups is especially important for postpartum recovery. The ball is also a great tool for improving pelvic-floor tone. Mothers have also commented that sitting on the ball with baby in arms is very soothing for the child, as it allows gentle, relaxing movement. Make sure you get a ball that comes with a hand pump. The package should cost about twenty dollars.

Hand Weights

Hand weights, or dumbbells, are useful when you are able to begin strength-training exercises. I recommend starting off with a set of five-, eight-, and ten-pound dumbbells. Hand weights come in many shapes and colors; stick to the less expensive brands. Look around; they should not cost you more than thirty dollars.

Mat

A mat is necessary for floor exercises. Find one that is padded. Mats are easy to store and are inexpensive, around fifteen dollars.

Exercise Bands

Exercise bands can be used in place of dumbbells for certain exercises.

The Program

The following stretching and strength-training suggestions should serve only as a guide as you work toward your fitness goals. Progress slowly and at your own rate. Kegels can be done the first day after labor. Stretching can be done daily as well; however, don't overstretch, and work up to the more complex stretches.

Kegel Exercises

When you were pregnant, no doubt you heard about Kegels. Kegel exercises, named after Dr. Arnold Kegel, were originally developed as a method for controlling incontinence in women following childbirth. It is now recommended that women do Kegel exercises during and after pregnancy to strengthen the muscles of the pelvic floor. These muscles, which support the urethra, bladder, uterus, and rectum, can weaken due to the excess weight of the baby and fluid. Kegel exercises can and should be done daily to strengthen these muscles and help prevent urine leakage. Kegels are also beneficial for toning the abdominals and lower back muscles.

To find these muscles, try stopping and starting the flow of urine. If you can do it, you've found the pelvic-floor muscles. Kegels can be done a few days after childbirth. The effort of doing these exercises daily is well worth the benefits. If you've been leaking a mild to moderate amount of urine following childbirth, chances are that doing Kegel exercises routinely will improve the situation, and perhaps even cure your incontinence. Try to make doing Kegels a habit during certain activities, such as feeding your baby, showering, or brushing your teeth, so you're reminded to do them each day. For the first four to six weeks following delivery, leaking a small amount of urine when you cough, laugh, or exert yourself is not abnormal. If leaking persists, it's a good idea to seek help from your doctor.

Kegel Exercises:

- Squeeze the pelvic-floor muscles, as if you're trying to stop the flow of urine.

• Tighten these muscles, holding for 10 seconds, then release. Repeat 15 to 25 times, 4 to 5 times per day.

Other Kegel Variations:

• Hold for 5 seconds, then relax, 12 to 15 times. Don't overdo it!

• While sitting in a chair, keep your feet slightly apart and your back straight. Tighten and relax your pelvic-floor muscles, holding for 5 seconds, then releasing.

• While sitting on the floor, keep your back flat against a wall and your legs extended in front of you with your feet slightly apart. To the count of 5, gradually tighten your pelvic-floor muscles, increasing tension with each count. Slowly release with each count to the starting position.

Stretching

Stretching is an important component to getting back to your prebaby shape. Gentle stretching is recommended immediately after birth, as long as you didn't have a complicated delivery. Stretching muscles of the lower and upper back and chest can help improve posture. You need to remember, however, that during pregnancy, estrogen and a substance called relaxin are released, which have the effect of relaxing ligaments, softening cartilage, and widening the pelvic joints due to an increase in synovial fluid. This fluid actually lubricates the joints of the body, which makes giving birth easier. Combined with other physiological effects, it can predispose you to injury when stretching and exercising if you are not careful. Deep, dynamic stretching is not recommended until the body starts to return to normal, about four to six weeks postpartum.

Try to stretch as many muscle groups as you can daily. If you've had a C-section, do gentle, static stretching and avoid putting too much strain on your abdominals. Never force a stretch; if you experience muscular pain during a stretch, you are pushing yourself too hard. Stretch to the point of mild discomfort and breathe deeply.

Recommended Stretches:

BACK AND SHOULDERS

LYING BACK BEND*

This stretch will help strengthen your back. Start slowly and don't force the stretch. Lie on your stomach with your arms at your sides, elbows bent, and hands at shoulder level, palms down. Slowly press your body up, keeping your hips touching the floor until you feel resistance in your lower back. Return to the floor; repeat 3 to 5 times.

STANDING BACK BEND*

Standing with your feet shoulder width apart, put hands on your lower back, breathe out slowly, arch your back, and look up at the ceiling. Don't go back too far; you should not feel any discomfort. Return to the beginning; repeat 3 to 5 times.

EXTENDED ARM STRETCH

Interlace your fingers in front of you at shoulder height. Turn your palms outward as you extend your arms forward to feel a stretch in your shoul-

*Not recommended following C-section

ders, middle of your upper back, arms, hands, fingers, and wrists. Hold for 10 to 12 seconds, then relax and repeat.

OVERHEAD ARM STRETCH

Interlace your fingers above your head. Turn your palms upward and push your arms slightly back and up. Feel the stretch in your arms, shoulders, and upper back. Hold for 10 to 12 seconds, then repeat. Make sure to breathe deeply.

SHOULDER/NECK STRETCH

To stretch the sides of your neck and tops of your shoulders, stand leaning your head sideways toward your left shoulder as your left hand pulls your right arm down and across, behind your back. Hold for 10 to 12 seconds; repeat on other side. Do each arm twice. This can also be done sitting on the floor or in a chair.

DELTOID STRETCH

Standing, reach your right arm across your chest, fully extended. Pushing your right elbow with your left hand, press your arm into your body. You should feel a stretch in the back of your shoulder, or posterior deltoid. Hold for 12 to 15 seconds, then release. Switch sides and stretch the left shoulder. Do each side twice.

TRICEPS STRETCH

Stand with your feet shoulder width apart. Your arms should be at your sides, palms facing backward. Raise your right arm and bring your forearm behind your head so that your elbow is at a 90-degree angle. Bring your left hand up and over the top of your head, gently pulling the right elbow to point vertically. Hold your head against your right elbow; your right hand should rest between your shoulder blades. You should feel a stretch along your right triceps. Hold for 12 to 15 seconds, then switch arms. Do each side twice.

STANDING SIDE STRETCH

Stand with your knees slightly bent, and raise your left elbow above your head. With your right hand, gently pull your left elbow behind your head as you bend your torso to the right. Hold an easy stretch for 10 seconds. Repeat on your right side. Keeping your knees bent will help your balance and prevent you from locking your knees.

BEHIND-THE-BACK STRETCH

Standing, raise your left arm over your head, then bend it so that your elbow points to the ceiling and your hand reaches down your back. Bend your right arm behind your back so that your elbow points to the floor and your hand, palm turned outward, reaches up your back toward your left hand. If you're able, grab the fingers of one hand with the other and hold. You may find that you can do one side of the stretch but not the other. Hold for 8 to 10 seconds, or as long as you feel comfortable, then repeat on the other side.

Variation

Dangle a towel behind your head with your right hand. With your right arm bent, reach up behind your back with your left hand to hold on to the dangling end of the towel. Gradually move your left hand up the towel, pulling your right arm down, until your hands are touching.

PRAYER STRETCH

Sitting on an excercise mat, place the soles of your feet together, letting your knees drop open to the sides. Reach forward, keeping your head down, and try to grab the front edge of the mat. Pulling with one arm isolates the stretch on either side. You should feel this in your shoulders. By slightly moving your hips in either direction, you can increase or decrease the stretch. Don't strain or try to reach farther than is comfortable. Hold for 10 to 12 seconds; repeat 2 to 3 times.

FOREARM AND WRIST STRETCH

Start on all fours. Turn your hands so that your fingers point backward, toward your knees. Keep palms flat as you move your hips backward to stretch the front part of your forearms. Hold for 15 seconds, relax, then repeat.

CAT STRETCH

Get on your hands and knees, with your back straight but relaxed. Exhale and walk your hands backward a few inches and arch your back up and forward into a cat pose. Hold for a count of 3, inhale, and relax. Repeat 3 times, adding more repetitions as you feel stronger.

SPINAL TWISTS

Sit on the floor and bend your left leg over your right knee so that your left knee points to the ceiling and your left foot rests on the floor on the outside of your right knee. Then, if it's comfortable, bend your right leg so that your right foot rests at the outside of your left knee. If you prefer, you may keep your right leg extended in front of you. Keeping your back straight, place your right hand on your left knee and use it as leverage to twist your body to the left. Twist so you can comfortably look over your left shoulder. Repeat on the opposite side. Hold 10 to 12 seconds.

KNEE TO CHEST STRETCH

Lying on your back, pull your right leg toward your chest. For this stretch, keep the back of your head on the floor. Repeat, pulling your left leg toward your chest. Be sure to keep your lower back flat and pressed into the floor. Do each leg twice.

STRETCHES FOR LEGS AND HIPS

LYING QUADRICEPS STRETCH

Lie on your left side and rest the side of your head in the palm of your left hand. Hold the top of your right foot between the toes and ankle with your right hand. Gently pull the right heel toward the right buttock to stretch the ankle and quads. Hold for 10 to 12 seconds, then repeat with the other leg. Do each leg 2 to 3 times.

STANDING QUADRICEPS STRETCH

Standing, maintain your balance by grabbing a chair, table, or wall in front of you with your right hand. Bend your left leg backward, holding the top of your left foot with your left hand. Keeping your knees together, bring your left heel to the back of your left buttock. Hold for 10 to 12 seconds, then repeat with the other leg. Do each leg twice.

BENT-LEG HAMSTRING STRETCH

Sitting on a mat, straighten your right leg out in front of you. Bend your left leg out to the side so that the sole of your left foot slightly touches the inside of your right thigh. Slowly bend forward from the hips toward the foot of the straight leg until you feel a slight stretch in your hamstring. Hold for 12 to 15 seconds. Switch sides and stretch the left leg in the same manner.

During this stretch, keep the foot of the straight leg upright with the ankle and toes relaxed. Be sure to keep the quadriceps relaxed. Do not dip your head forward when initiating the stretch.

If you cannot easily reach your ankle or foot with your outstretched hands, sling a towel around the sole of your foot, holding the ends in either hand, and pull on the towel to help you stretch forward.

LYING HAMSTRING STRETCH

Lie flat on your back on a mat or carpeted floor. Lift your left leg up perpendicular to the floor. Your right leg should be flat on the floor. Interlock your hands behind your left knee, pulling your leg toward your chest until you feel a stretch in your left hamstring. Hold for 12 to 15 seconds, then repeat with the opposite leg. Do each leg twice.

HIPS AND GROIN STRETCH

Sit with your legs stretched out straight in front of you, a comfortable distance apart. To stretch the inside of your upper legs and hips, slowly lean forward from your hips. Be sure to keep your quadriceps relaxed and your feet upright. Hold for 15 to 20 seconds. Keep your hands out in front of you for balance and stability. *Do not* lean forward with your head and shoulders. This will cause your hips to move backward and put pressure on your lower back.

The Exercise Plan

The following exercises are recommended if you've had a normal, straightforward birth. Keep it simple; don't overdo it. If you tire, rest and start again the next day. Listen to your body. Some women will be able to advance more quickly than others. The exercises are outlined by days and weeks. Don't be too concerned about the week; progress as you feel comfortable. Veteran moms just starting an exercise program may start farther into the program (about week 3).

Days 1, 2, and 3—
Yes, you may feel up to it!

PELVIC-FLOOR EXERCISES

KEGELS (SEE PAGES 46–47)

You can do these while lying in bed. Slowly contract your pelvic-floor muscles and hold for 5 seconds, then slowly release. Repeat 5 to 10 times. Over time, increase repetitions to 50 to 75 per day.

ABDOMINALS

ABDOMINAL TIGHTENING

This very simple exercise can be done in bed, and promotes the process of abdominal healing. Starting this the first few days after labor will help get your abs back to their old shape.

Lying on your back, suck in your abdominals and hold for 3 to 5 seconds. Release. During the first week, gradually work up to 5 seconds. Do 8 to 10 repetitions and 2 to 3 sets daily.

PELVIC TILTS

Lying on your back with knees bent, inhale and suck in your abdomen, pulling in through your belly button. Tighten your buttocks and slowly flatten the small of your back. Hold this position 3 to 5 seconds then slowly exhale. Gradually increase the hold to 5 seconds and progress to doing one exercise 8 to 10 times a day by the tenth day.

DEEP BREATHING

Deep abdominal breathing will help you regain strength in your abdominal muscles, and it promotes healing. Each time you take a deep breath, you get oxygen throughout your body while also reinflating your lungs.

Lying in bed, bend your knees (if able). Relax your body, allowing your weight to sink into the surface of the bed. Put your hands on your abdomen, close your eyes, and be aware of your breathing. Inhale; you will feel your abdomen and hands rise. Stretch your abdominal muscles outward. Hold for a count of 5. Exhale, pulling in your abdominal muscles. Hold for another count of 5. Repeat 3 to 5 times, progressing to doing one repetition 10 times a day by the end of the first week.

ANKLE CIRCLES (TO ENHANCE CIRCULATION)

Make 8 to 10 circles with your ankles clockwise, then repeat counterclockwise. Repeat circular pattern 3 to 5 times. Do the ankle circles in different positions, such as lying, sitting, etc.

Remainder of the First Week

After the first couple of days, you may feel up to a walk. Some women are able to take a walk while still in the hospital. Just take it slowly and have help nearby.

Stretching is also important. Try to do a couple of easy stretches as recommended earlier in this section.

Exercises for Week 2

CARDIOVASCULAR

Most moms will find walking the only form of aerobic exercise they can do at this stage. Try to take three 5- to 10-minute walks in week 2, if you're physically able.

Add these to the previous exercises and stretches:

ABDOMINALS

LEG SLIDES

Lying on your back, bend your right leg, keeping your foot flat on the floor. Start with your left leg extended on the floor, then tilt your pelvis up to keep your lower back flat as you slide your left heel up and down on the floor. Work only the range where you can keep your lower back flat on floor. Repeat with other leg. Make sure to keep your abs pressed into the floor throughout. Do 2 sets of 8 to 10 repetitions.

HEAD-UPS (NOT RECOMMENDED IF YOU HAVE A DIASTASIS)

Lie on your back with knees bent and arms crossed over your chest or at your sides. Breathe in. Slowly breathe out and raise your head until you can see your knees. Hold for a count of 3. Slowly lower your head. Repeat 3 to 5 times, every 4 hours, increasing to 25 to 30 head-ups a day at the end of the week.

Do You Have a Diastasis?

Before doing more advanced abdominal exercises, it is important to check for extensive separation of the abdominal muscles, or *diastasis*. The recti muscles fan out on both sides of a central seam that runs from the breastbone to the pubic bone. During pregnancy, these muscles may separate noticeably. Crunches, sit-ups, and other abdominal exercises can worsen the problem. How to check yourself:

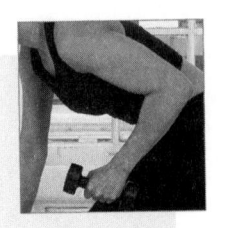

- Lie on your back with your knees bent, feet flat on floor, and pelvis in a neutral alignment.
- Put one hand behind your head.
- Raise your head and place your first two fingers of the other hand on your abdomen in line with your belly button.
- Press down gently into the soft gap between the two firm recti muscles. A one-to-two-inch, finger-width gap is normal. If the gap is larger, you may have a diastasis.

EXERCISES FOR A DIASTASIS

LEG SLIDES (SEE PAGE 57)

As your strength allows, add the following exercises:

V-UPS

Lie on your back with your knees bent, feet flat on floor, and pelvis in a neutral alignment. Put your hands on your abdomen, forming two V's that don't touch. As you lift your head slightly off the floor, tighten your abs. Push down and in with your fingers to push the two sides of the abdominal muscles together. Start with 3 sets of 5 repetitions. Gradually build to 12 to 15 repetitions.

TOWEL CRUNCH

Lie on your back with your knees bent, feet flat on floor, and pelvis in a neutral position. Wrap a towel or sheet around your midsection. This will act as a splint. Cross the ends of the towel below your belly button. Lift your head a few inches off the floor, tightening your abs and pulling the two ends of the towel together. Start with 3 to 5 repetitions and gradually build up to 3 sets of 10 to 12 repetitions.

After 3 to 4 weeks, the gap should not be noticeable. If it is, speak to your doctor.

LOWER-BACK EXERCISES

Over half of women report lower-back pain during postpartum recovery. This is due to an increased strain on the muscles, ligaments, and joints of the body during pregnancy from posture changes as the baby grows and ligaments loosen due to hormonal softening effects.

HUGGIES

Lie flat on your back, knees bent and feet raised. Hug your knees and at the same time bring your chin to your chest. Tilt your pelvis to make sure your lower back is flat. Breathe in. Slowly breathe out and return to starting position. Repeat 3 to 5 times, gradually increasing to 10 times a day.

BALL EXERCISES

This can be done with or without a diastasis. Sit on a fitness ball, back straight and feet flat on floor. Keep your abdominals tight. This simple activity will improve your posture and help begin the process of healing and tightening the abs.

Exercises for Week 3

The three-week point may be a good place for veteran moms to start if they are just beginning an exercise program. Make sure to get the okay from your doctor first.

CARDIOVASCULAR

By week 3, some women are able to start some of the cardio options that they enjoyed while they were pregnant. See pages 38 through 40 for cardio recommendations. When increasing your cardio, it's important to check your heart rate frequently in order to ensure you are staying in the lower portion of your target heart rate zone (page 43). Make sure your heart rate does not go above 150 beats per minute.

Continue doing the previous exercises from weeks 1 and 2. Add more of the recommended stretches before and after your program. Begin to add more of the following as your strength allows:

UPPER BODY

TRICEPS EXTENSION—OVERHEAD

(Targets triceps)

Sitting on a stable bench or ball, keep your knees bent and your feet flat on the floor. Holding one dumbbell, bring it behind your head, keeping your elbow close to your ear. Keeping your abdominals tight, slowly straighten your arm to full extension, being careful not to lock your elbow. Lower your arm to the starting position and repeat. Repeat exercise with your other arm. Start with 8 repetitions, gradually building up to 2 sets of 8 to 10 repetitions.

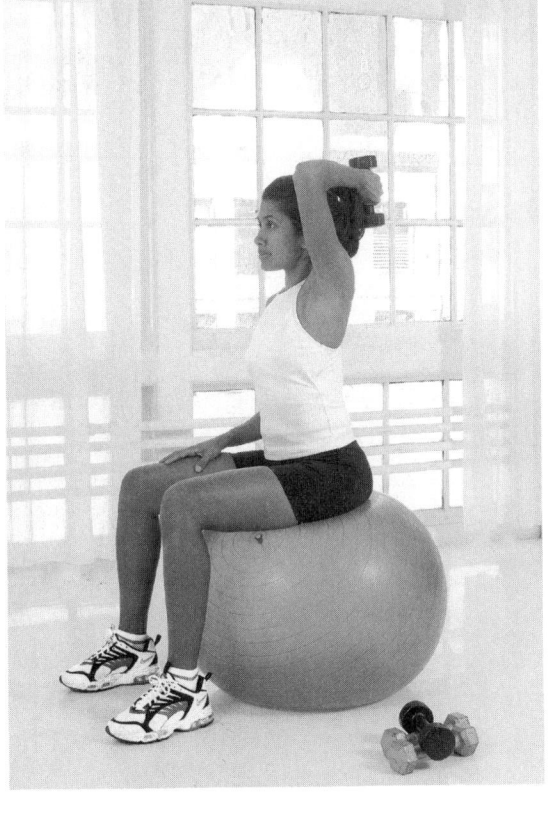
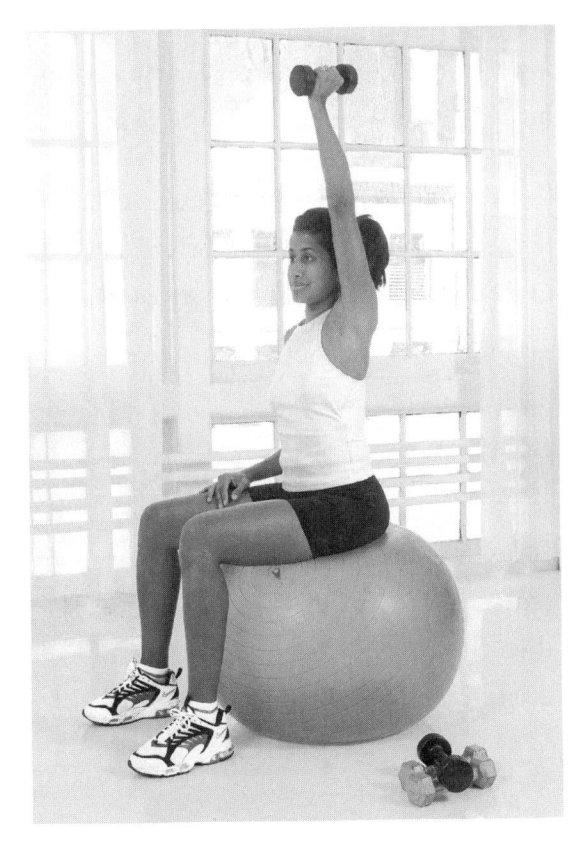

ABDOMINALS

Do these exercises *only* if the gap in your abdominal muscles has closed.
If not, continue with the modified exercises described earlier.

CURL-UPS

Lying on your back, bend your knees and put both feet on the ground. Put your hands on your thighs. Exhale, contract your abdominals, and lift your head and shoulders off the ground. As you do this, slide your hands toward your knees. Try to get your shoulder blades off the ground. Hold this position for a count of 5, then slowly roll down to the starting position. Relax. Start with 6 to 8 repetitions the first day, then gradually increase to 2 sets of 8 to 12.

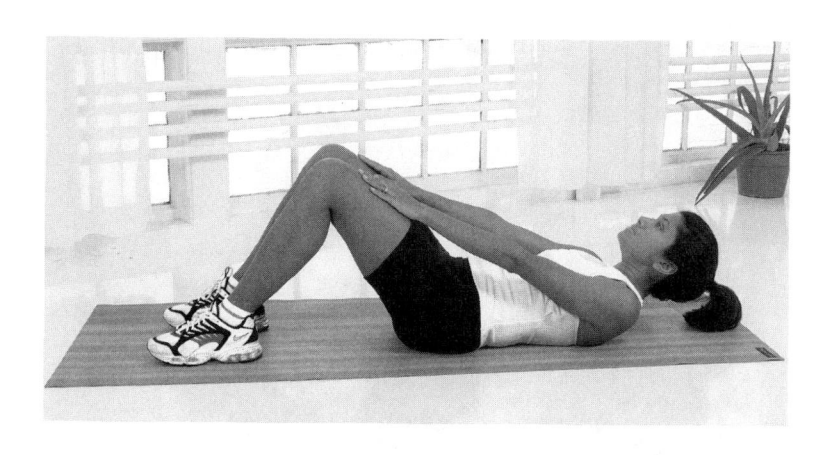

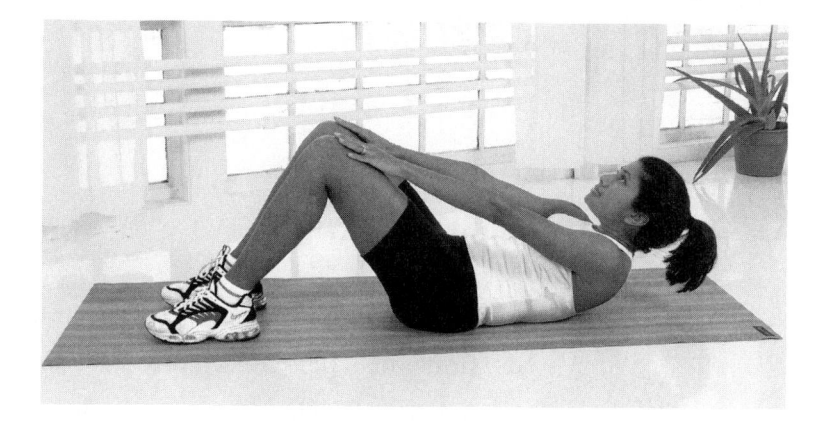

DIAGONAL CURL-UPS

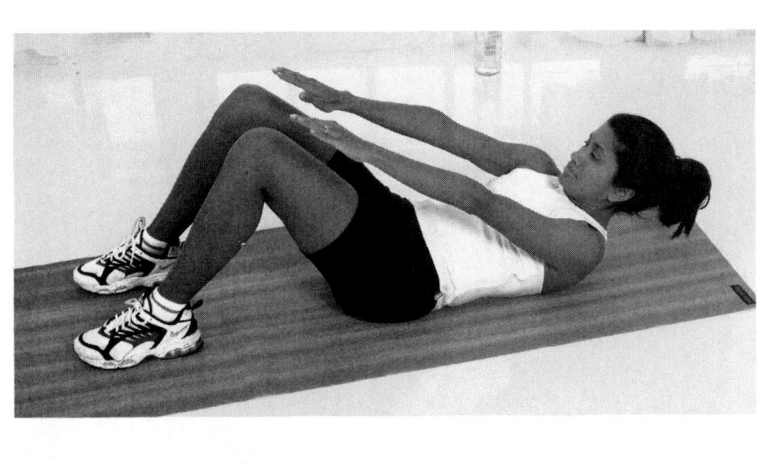

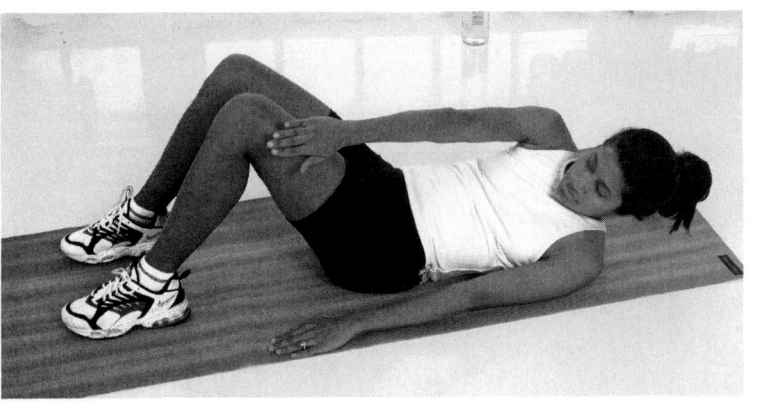

Lying on your back, bend your knees and put both feet on the ground. Your arms should be reaching toward your knees. As you breathe out, slowly curl up, reaching diagonally. Reach your right hand to the outside of your left knee. Repeat on the other side. Start with 4 to 6 repetitions the first day, gradually increasing to 8 to 12. As you become stronger, lift your knee to the opposite elbow with your hands clasped behind your head.

MODIFIED PLANK

Kneeling, place your forearms on the ground, shoulder width apart. Inch your arms forward, keeping your back as straight as possible. Pull your abdominals in and tighten them as you form a plank. Start with trying to hold the plank 3 to 5 seconds. As you become stronger, try to do a set of 3, holding for 10 to 12 seconds.

LOWER BACK

SUPER MOMS

Lying facedown on a mat, extend your legs, toes pointed. Extend your arms over your head. Look forward, keeping your head steady and your chin off the ground. Slowly raise your right arm and left leg at the same time until they are a few inches off the ground. Slowly lower to starting position. Repeat with your left arm and right leg. Start with 8 to 10 repetitions for each arm and leg. Gradually build up to 2 to 3 sets, 10 to 12 repetitions.

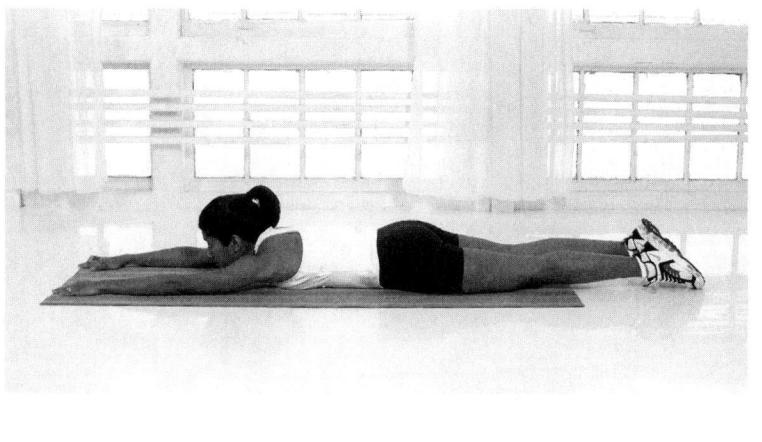

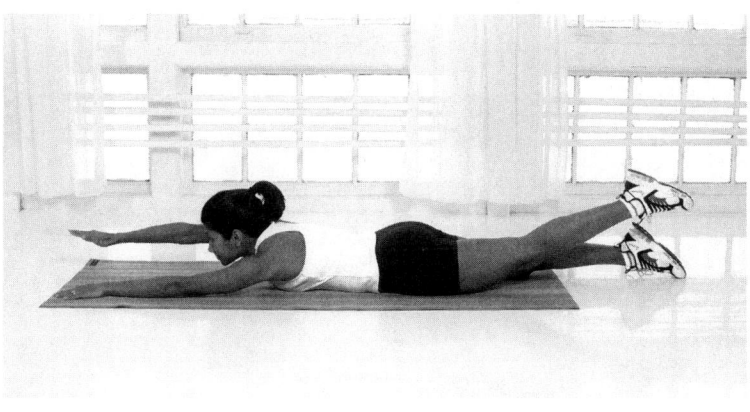

BALL EXERCISES

BRIDGE ABDOMINALS, LOWER BACK
(NOT RECOMMENDED IF YOU HAVE A DIASTASIS)

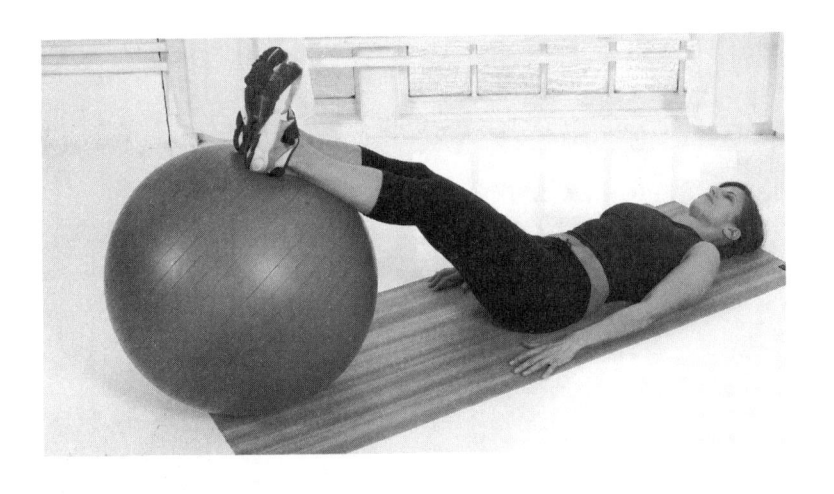

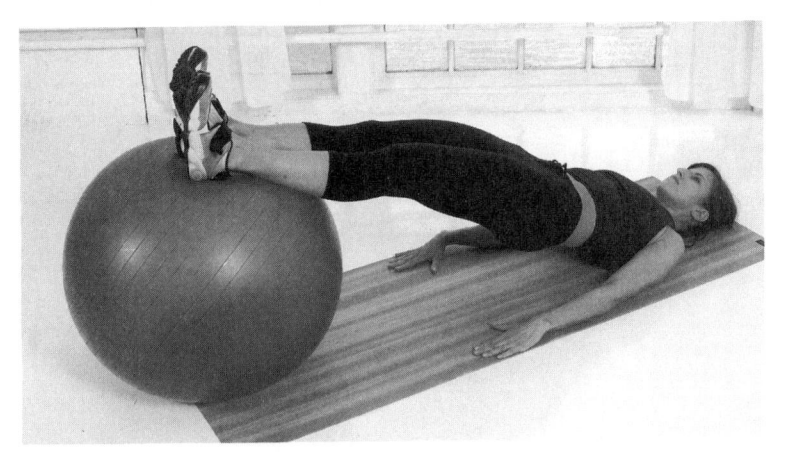

Lie faceup on an exercise mat or carpeted floor with your arms in a relaxed position at your sides. Place your feet on the ball so that the ball is just resting under your lower legs. Raise your pelvis off the floor by tightening the buttock muscles so that the body forms a straight diagonal line from shoulders to feet. Hold this position 5 to 10 seconds; repeat. Gradually build up to 2 sets of 8 to 10 repetitions.

Exercises for Weeks 4 and 5

CARDIOVASCULAR

If you're feeling strong at the four-week point, increase your aerobic workouts to fifteen to twenty minutes. If you can't find a solid twenty minutes, break it down into two sets of ten minutes. Keep in mind your ligaments may still be loose for at least three months following childbirth, so avoid any high-impact exercises or sports that require quick changes of direction. Deep, dynamic stretching should also be avoided. As long as you get the okay from your doctor, you should be able to start the following cardiovascular activities:

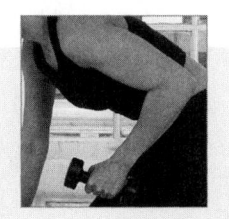

- **BRISK WALKING ALTERNATING WITH JOGGING**
- **SWIMMING**
- **YOGA**
- **LOW-IMPACT AEROBICS**
- **BIKING**
- **STRENGTH TRAINING**

Make sure you begin each workout with at least five minutes of warm-up and stretching, followed by a cool-down.* If you had a diastasis, it should be healed after four weeks. Be sure to check with your doctor if it hasn't and don't do any of the strenuous abdominal exercises.

 *Carefully monitor your pulse, making sure you are staying in your target heart rate.

You may continue to do the exercises that you did during the previous weeks, gradually building on sets and repetitions. Don't forget to do your Kegels; your pelvic floor is still recovering!

Some of the following exercises will start to incorporate free weights and more intensity. This program has proven successful for new moms trying to regain their prebaby shape as well as for the veteran mom just starting an exercise program. Improving your upper and lower body strength is especially important now that you are carrying a ten-to-fifteen-pound infant around: the added weight can put a strain on your lower back. If you're a beginner, start with one set and gradually build up to two to three sets of ten to twelve repetitions. Start with light weights, three to five pounds, and gradually increase the weight as you get stronger. Both concentric (bringing the weight toward your body) and eccentric (pushing the weight away from your body) phases should be done to slow counts of four. Remember, you are still in recovery—don't push it! If you feel tired or you exceed your target heart rate, stop and wait until the next day.

UPPER BODY

Try to do one of each muscle group, every other day.

MODIFIED PUSH-UPS—NO BALL

(Targets pectoralis and triceps muscles)

From a kneeling position, place your hands flat on the ground, shoulder width apart. There should be a direct line from your shoulder to the middle of your hand. Bend your elbows and lower your chest to the floor.

Keep your head steady, looking straight down toward the floor. Return to the starting position. To increase the intensity, lift one knee off the ground, keeping your weight balanced on one knee and your hands.

ALTERNATING ARM RAISES (CAN BE DONE STANDING OR WHILE SITTING ON A FITNESS BALL)

(Targets anterior deltoids)

Standing on one foot, hold a dumbbell in each hand, palms facing your body and resting on your thighs. Keep your knees slightly bent, feet shoulder width apart. With your right arm, slowly raise the dumbbell to shoulder height, pause, then lower to starting position. Repeat, switching arms and standing leg.

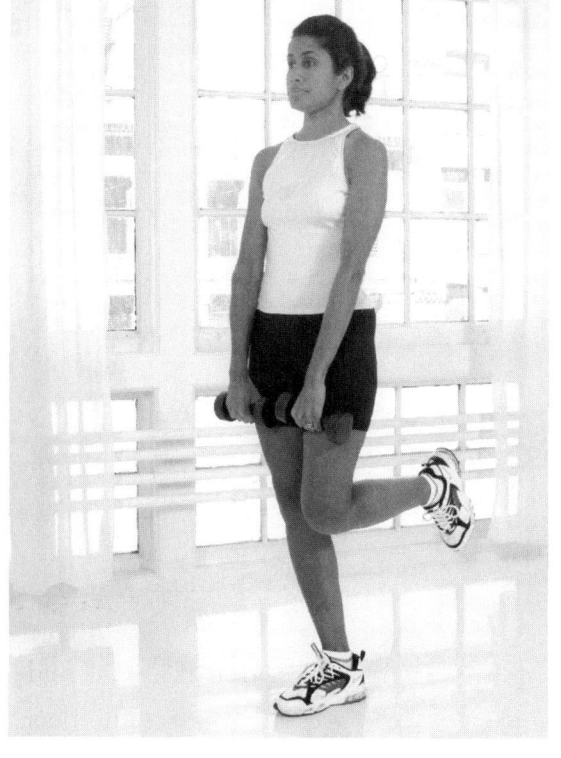
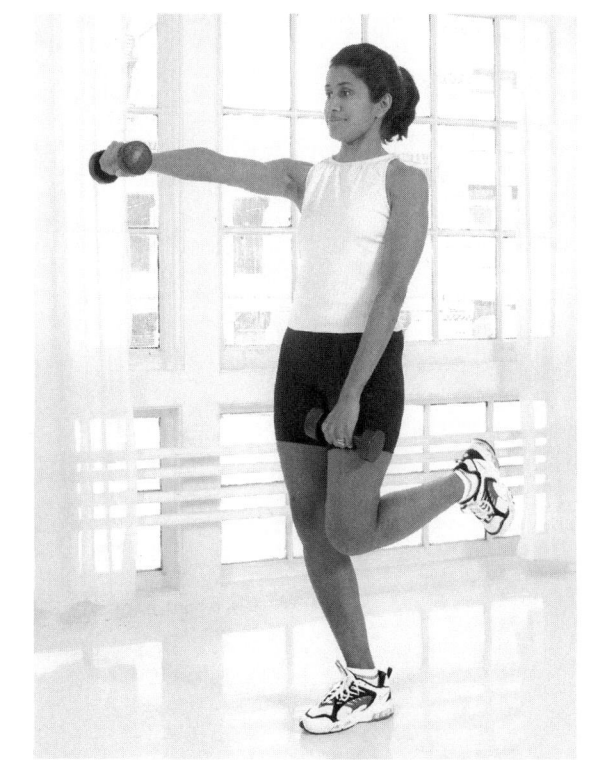

ALTERNATING BICEPS CURLS—ONE FOOT

(Targets biceps, forearms, and improves core strength)

Standing on one foot, hold a dumbbell in each hand, arms at your sides, palms facing in. Keep your back straight and your feet shoulder width apart. Slowly curl the right dumbbell up toward your right biceps, slowly turning your wrist so your palm is facing your shoulder. Aim to keep your elbows tucked at your sides, and avoid swinging the weights up or arching your back. Lower to the starting position, turning your wrist so your palm is facing in at the end of the curl. Keeping your abdominals and buttocks tight throughout the motion will help you balance on one foot. Repeat with left arm, switching feet.

EXERCISES WITH BALL FOR UPPER BODY

FLY

**(Targets the minor and major pectorals as well as
the front of the deltoids)**

Lie with the ball under your shoulders, feet shoulder width apart. Your
head and neck should be stabilized on the ball. Hold a dumbbell in each
hand and extend your arms out at chest height with your palms facing inward. Keep your elbows soft; do not lock them. Slowly lower the dumbbells out to the sides, forming an arc, but do not let your arms fall below
shoulder level, as this places too much strain on the shoulders. When
you feel a pull in the shoulders, slowly return your arms back to the starting position, forming an arc on the way up.

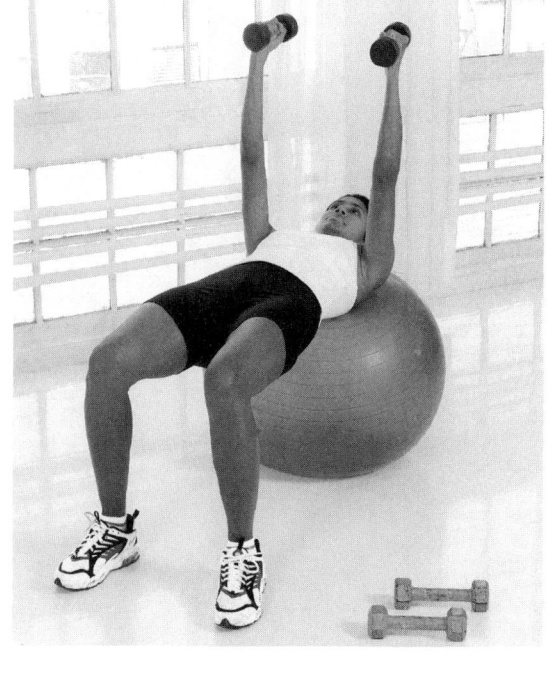
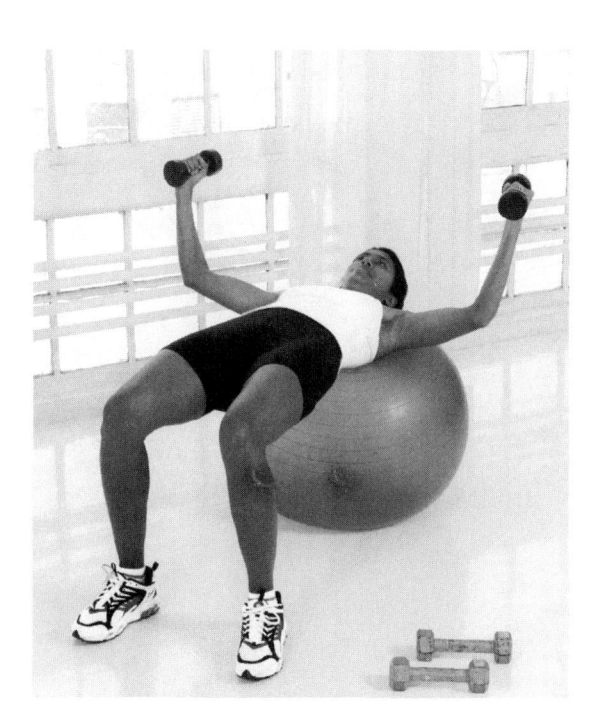

TRICEPS EXTENSION

(Targets all parts of triceps)

Stand with your right hand and knee firmly on the ball and your left leg slightly flexed so that your torso is nearly parallel to the floor. Hold a dumbbell in your left hand with your elbow flexed at a 90-degree angle and your palm facing inward. Try to keep your back as flat as possible. Keeping your elbow pressed into your side, use your forearm to slowly move the dumbbell backward until your arm is straight. Hold for 3 seconds and return to the starting position. Repeat with other arm.

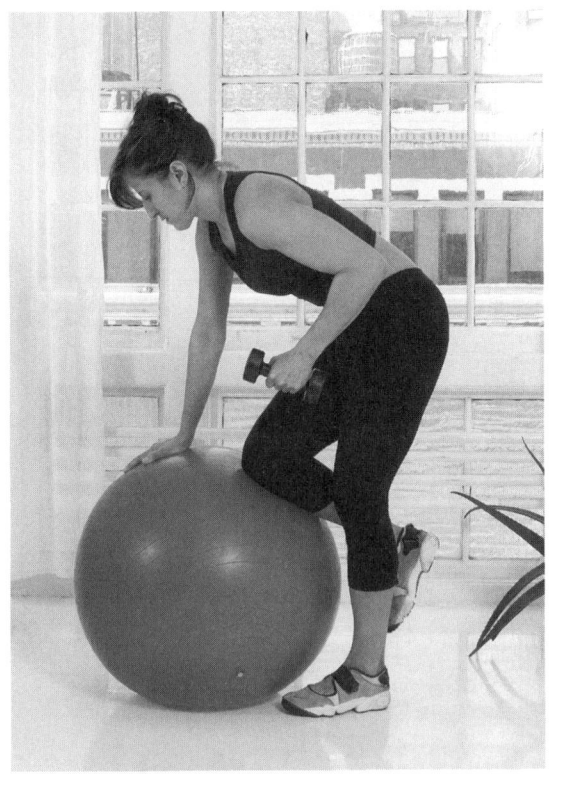 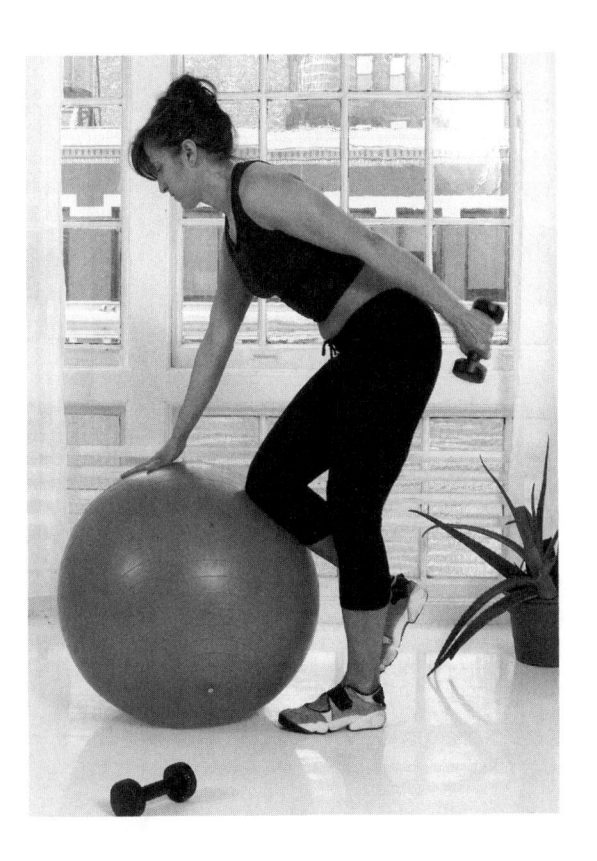

LOWER BODY, PELVIS, AND BACK

Try to do one of the exercises every day. Make sure not to do the same muscle group two days in a row

LUNGES

(Targets the quadriceps, buttocks)

Standing, place your feet shoulder width apart. Hold a dumbbell in each hand, palms facing in. Keep your abdominals tight. With your left foot, take a step forward. Your right leg should be almost straight. Slowly lower your body by bending your left leg. Be sure to keep the left knee over the left toe. Just before your right knee touches the ground, slowly push up to the starting position. Start by repeating for one set, then switch legs.

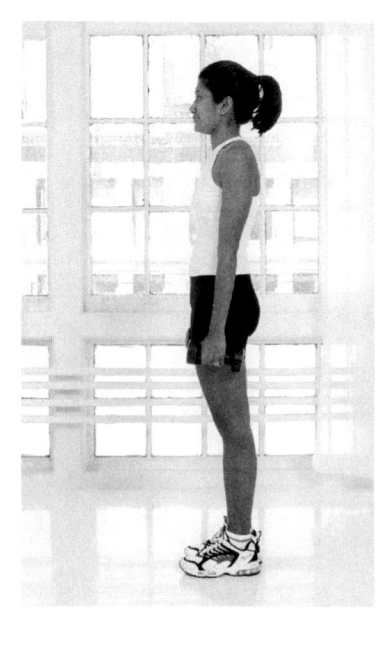 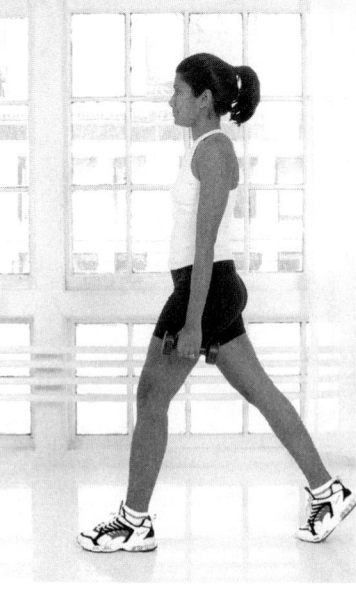 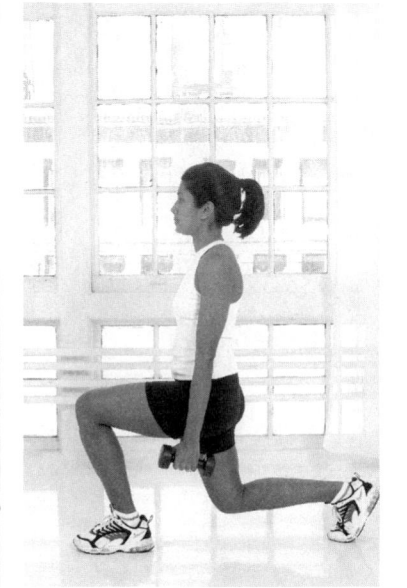

DUMBBELL SQUATS

(Targets the quadriceps, buttocks)

Hold a dumbbell between your knees. Slightly pronate (turn out) your feet. Keeping your elbows slightly bent, lower your body, bending at the knees until your thighs are parallel to the floor. Be sure to keep your back straight, head looking straight ahead. Pause, then slowly return to the starting position.

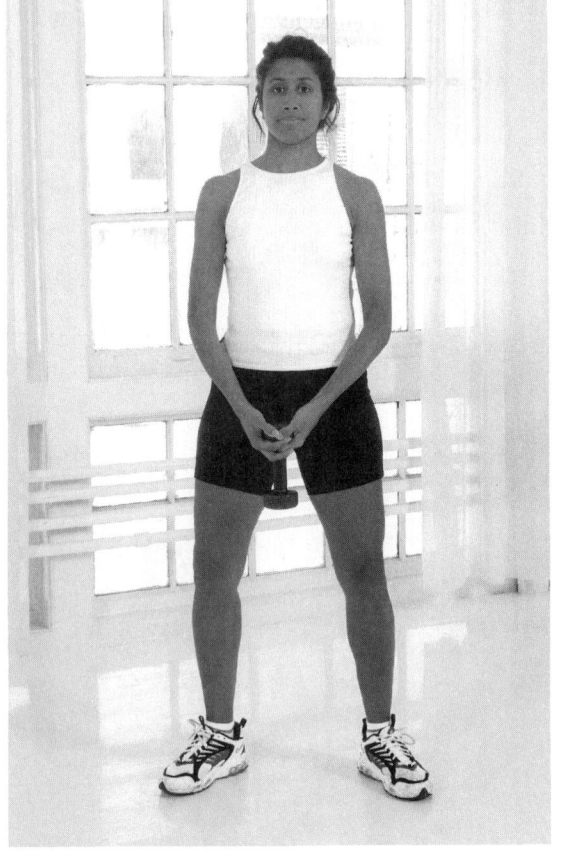
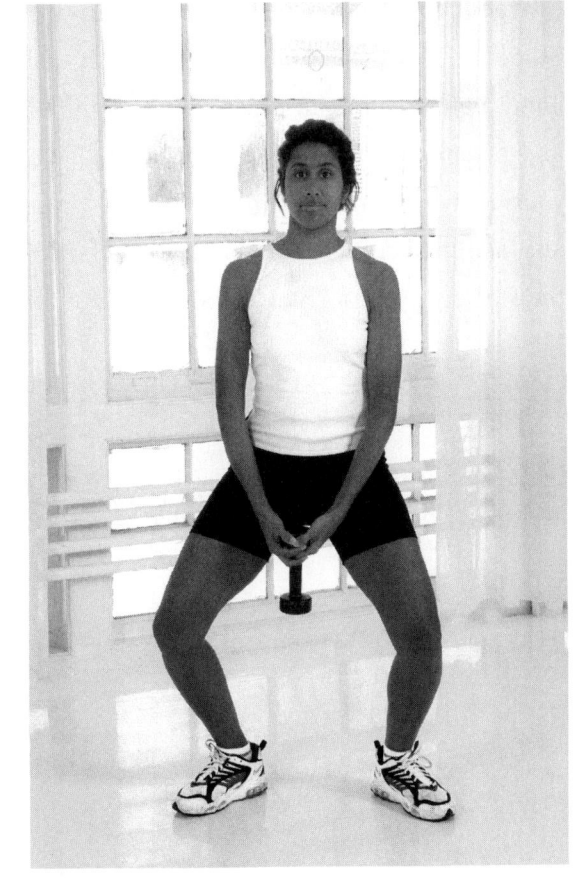

CALF RAISES

(Targets the gastrocnemius muscle [calf])
Stand with your feet together, holding a dumbbell in each hand. Palms should be facing in, resting on the sides of your legs. Slowly, raise up to your tiptoes (as high as you can), keeping your ankles stable. Pause for 3 seconds, then lower to the starting position.

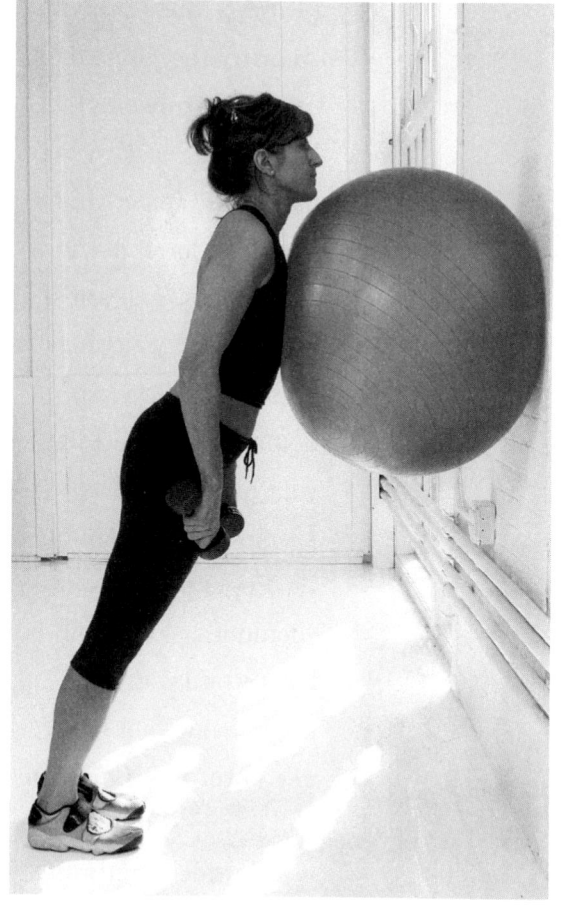 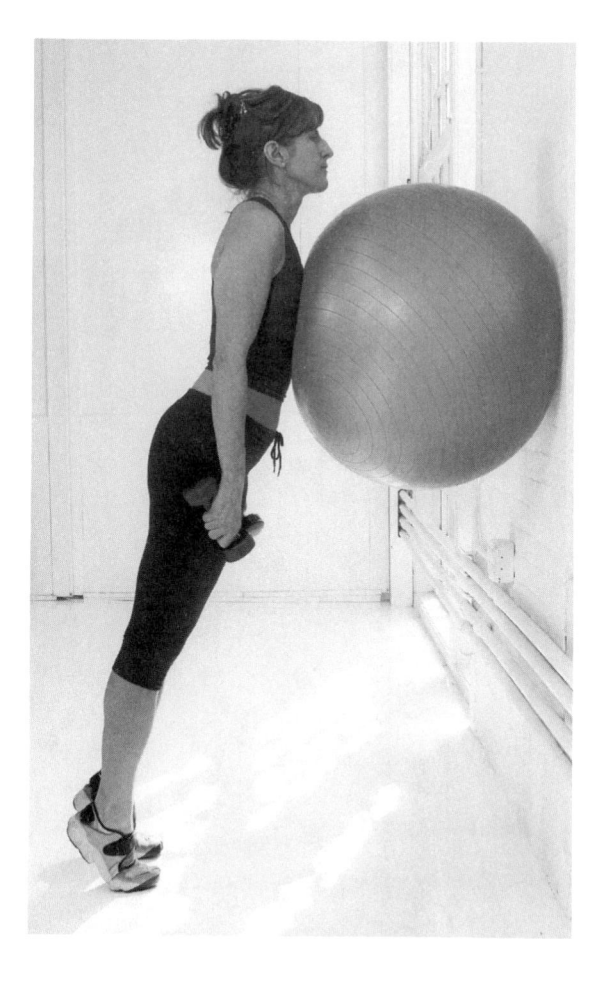

EXERCISES WITH BALL FOR LOWER BODY

Pick out at least two different muscle groups each day.

LEG CURLS

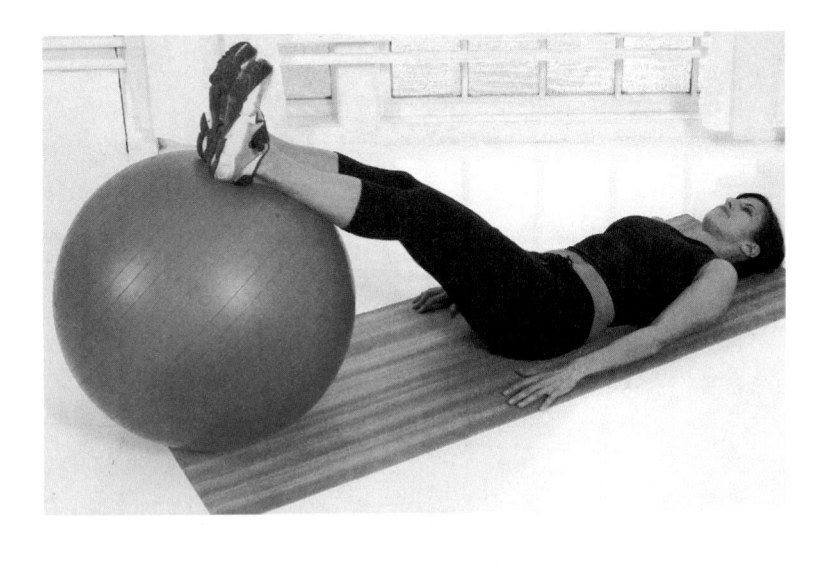

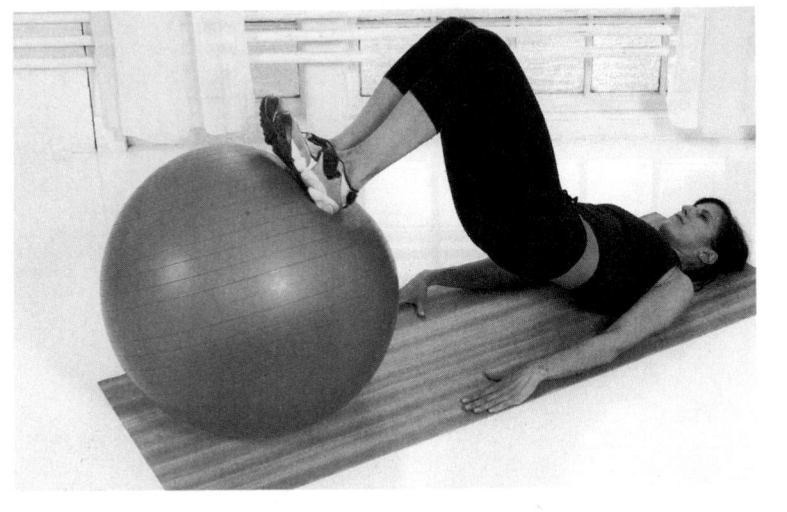

(Targets the hamstrings, buttocks, and calf muscles)
Lie on your back with a ball placed under your heels and lower portion of your legs. Your arms should be at your sides. Tighten the lower abdominal muscles. Lift your hips and pelvis, keeping your weight on the upper part of your shoulders. Slowly roll the ball toward your buttocks, using your heels and lower legs. Once the ball is almost touching your buttocks, return to the starting position. Keep your hips lifted throughout the set.

HIP EXTENSIONS

(Targets the pelvis and quadriceps)

Kneel on the floor with the ball under your chest and tighten your abdominal muscles. Slowly extend your right arm and left leg until they are in a straight line with your hip, knee, and toe. Hold for 3 seconds and return to the starting position. Repeat using the left arm and right leg.

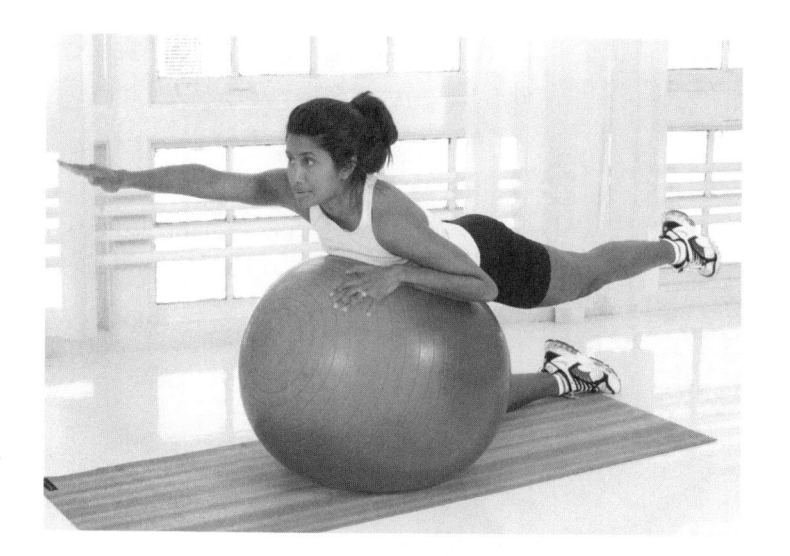

HIP FLEXION

(Targets the hip flexors)

Lie with the ball under your abdominals and roll forward until the ball is below your knees. Tighten your lower abs and keep your back straight. Slowly bring your knees to your chest, using the hip flexors to bring the ball in. Hold for 3 seconds, then slowly roll to the starting position.

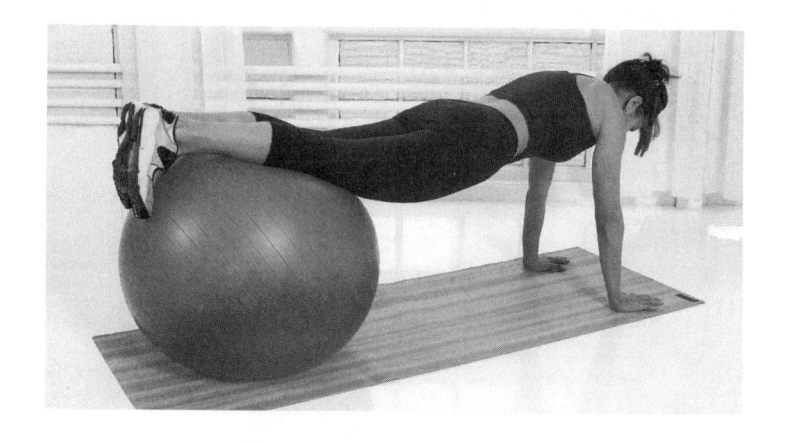

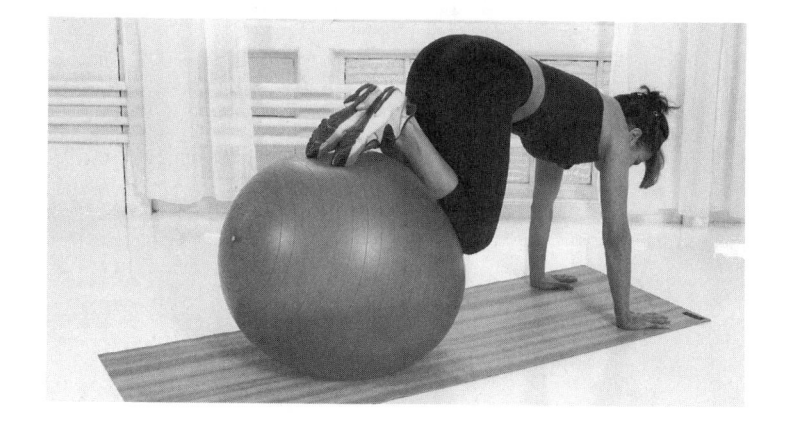

LUNGES—DO EITHER LUNGES OR SQUATS, EVERY OTHER DAY

(Targets the quadriceps)

Stand with a ball under your right shin and bend your left knee slightly. Keeping your back straight, lunge forward so the left leg is in a semi-squat position and the right leg is extended on the ball. Hold for a few seconds then straighten the left leg to the starting position. Start with one set then repeat with the other leg.

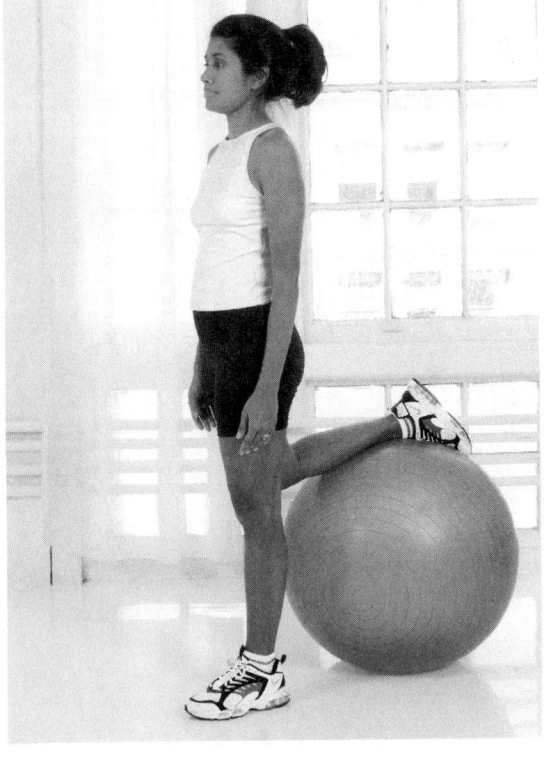
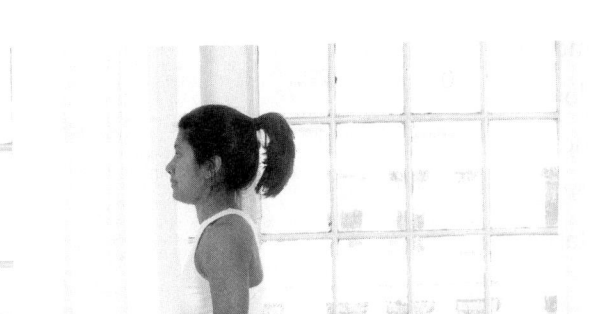

LYING SIDE RAISE

(Targets the adductor and abductor muscles)
Lie on your side and place an exercise ball between your feet. Keeping your abdominals tight and your back straight, slowly lift the ball a few inches off the ground. Pause, then lower to the starting position.

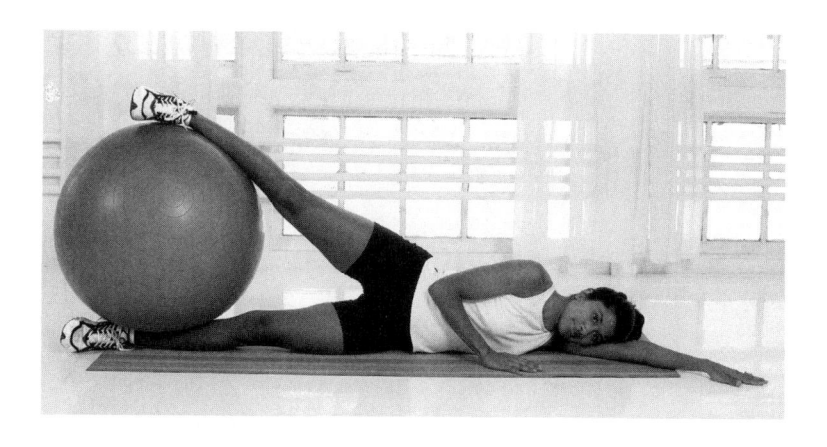

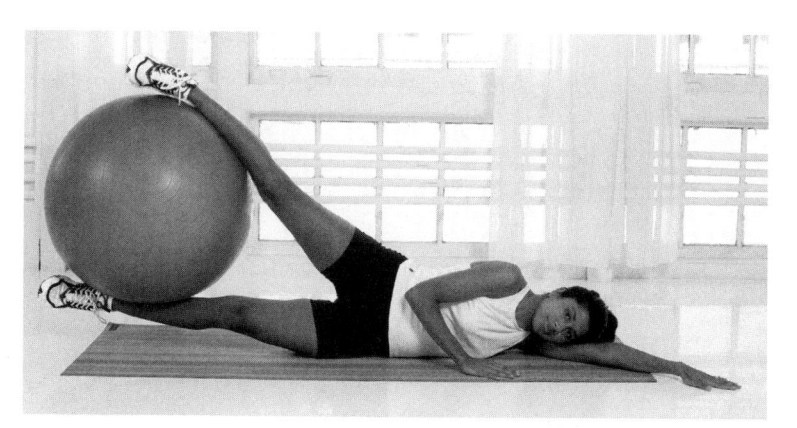

ABDOMINALS

Most of the abdominal exercises I recommend are done on the ball. Try to do two of each every day.

PLANK—WITHOUT BALL

(Targets lower abdominals, lower back)
Lie facedown on an exercise mat, supported by your elbows directly under your shoulders and your flexed toes on the mat. Place one hand on

top of the other so your forearms form a triangle. Tighten your abdominals and lift your entire body so it is now as straight as a plank and supported by your toes and elbows.

SITTING CRUNCH

(Targets the rectus abdominis)

Lie with a ball under the middle of your back and place your feet flat on the ground, shoulder width apart. Place your hands behind your head, thumbs below your earlobes. Your hands are used to stabilize your head, not pull it up. Slowly lift your shoulders forward and keep your head straight, focusing on the ceiling. Lift about 3 to 4 inches or until you feel your abs contract, then lower to the starting position. Start with one set of 10.

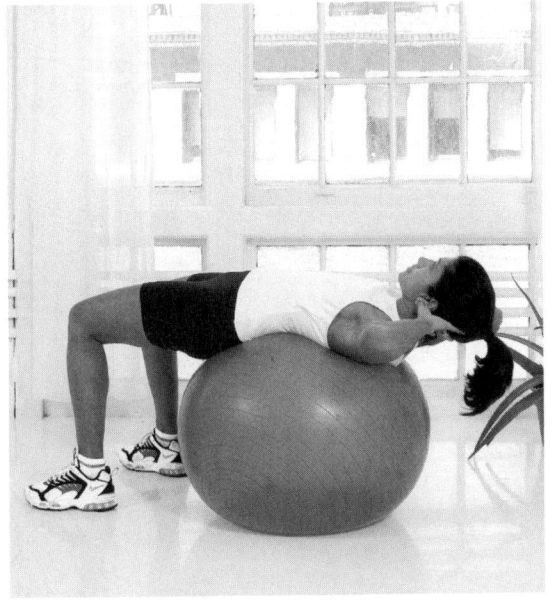 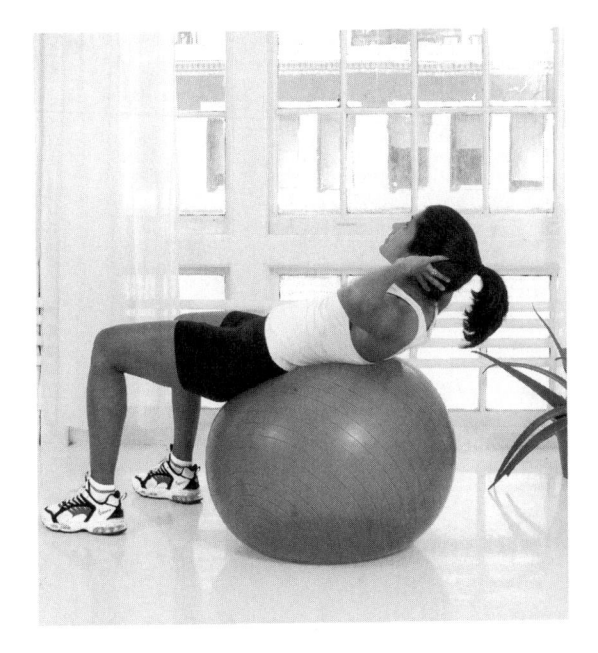

CRUNCH WITH FEET ON BALL

(Targets the rectus abdominis)

Lying on your back, place both your heels on a ball, keeping your hips and knees at a 90-degree angle. Place your hands behind your head, thumbs below your earlobes. Your hands are used to stabilize, not to pull, your neck. Tighten your abdominals and lift your shoulders from the floor toward your knees. Hold, then lower to the starting position. Start with a set of 8 to 10.

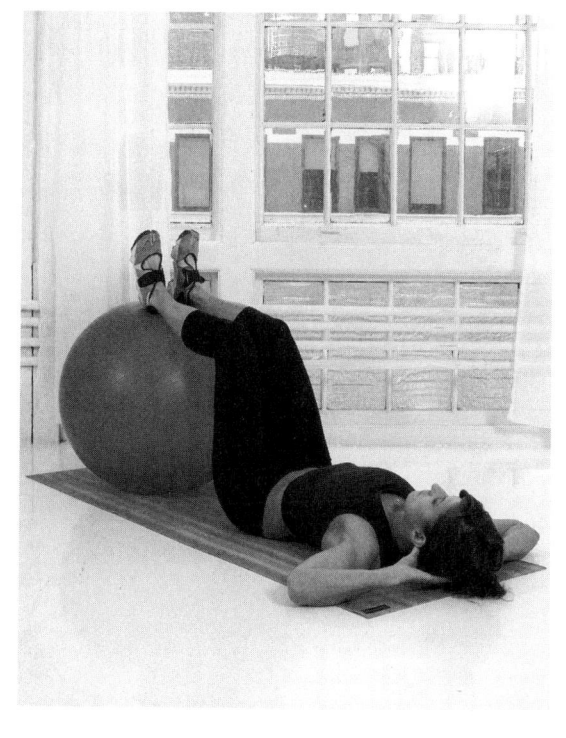
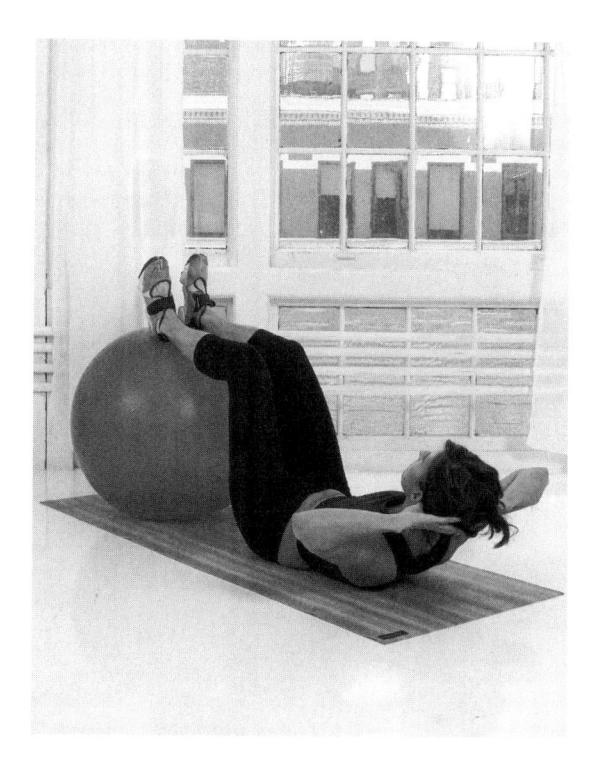

REVERSE CRUNCH

(Targets the upper rectus abdominis)

Lie on the floor and grasp the ball under your knees. Lift the ball up from the floor. Place your hands behind your head, thumbs under your earlobes. Hands should be used to stabilize, not to pull, the neck. Slowly lift your shoulders from the floor toward your knees. Pause, then return your upper body to the starting position. The ball remains lifted, under your knees. Start with one set of 8 to 10 repetitions.

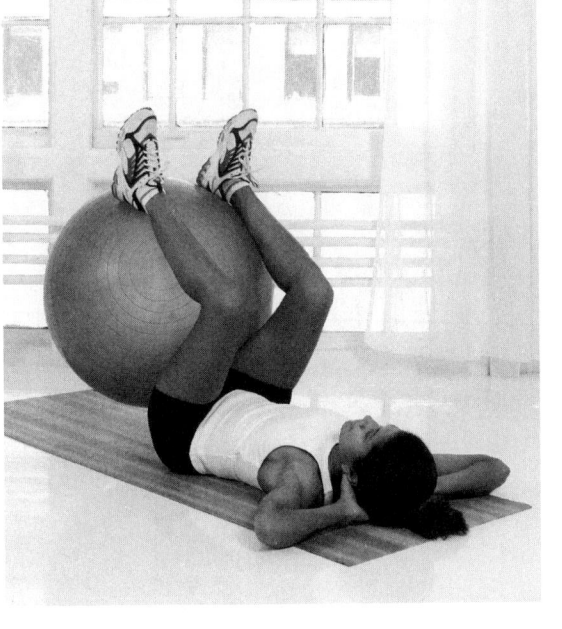
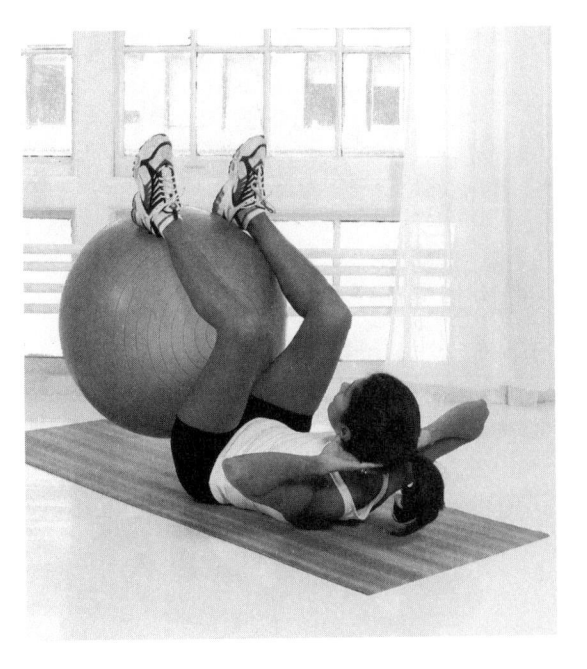

OBLIQUES

(Targets the external obliques)

Lie on the floor with the ball under your heels. Your hips and knees should be at a 90-degree angle. As you tighten your abdominals, reach down to the left side, trying to touch the side of the ball. Be careful not to arch your back. Pause, return to the starting position. Repeat on the right side. Start with one set of 8 to 10 repetitions.

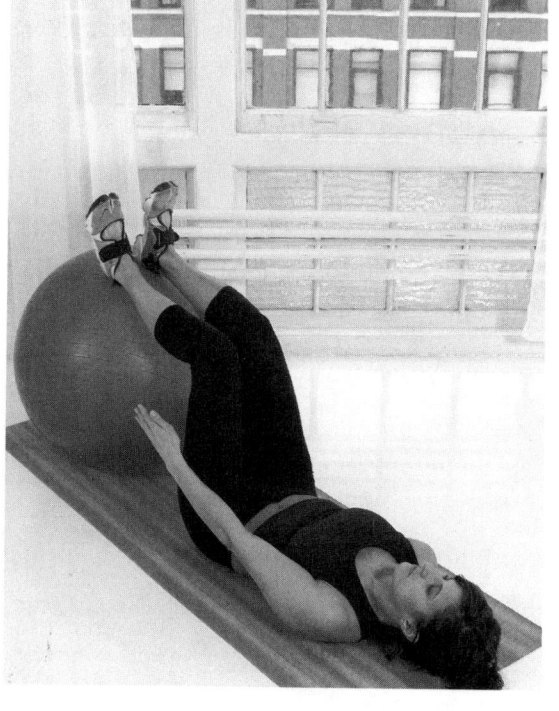 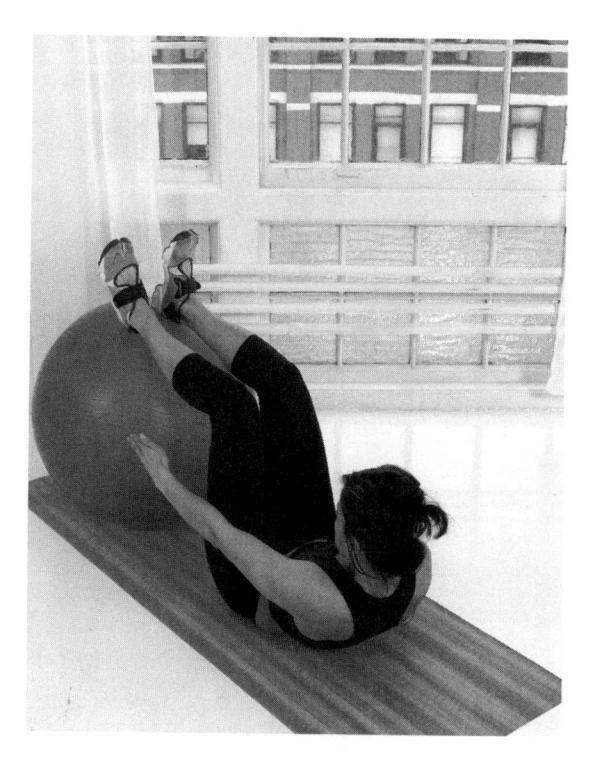

Exercises for Weeks 6 and Beyond

Congratulations! You've made it to six weeks postpartum! Now is the point where you can step up your workouts and go at them with full intensity. Discuss your program with your doctor at your six-week checkup. Most women are concerned about their abdominals at the six-week point, as they may not be back to their prebaby shape. Focus now on more intense abdominal work, as well as strengthening muscles of the lower back and pelvis. The lower back and pelvis need to be supported and stabilized to protect the lower spine from being injured when you're lifting, moving, and carrying objects. The exercises I recommend will help strengthen such core muscles. Remember, it takes at least eight weeks after childbirth for the abdominal muscles to effectively stabilize the pelvis and protect the spine.

Perhaps you've been working out and making smart food choices but still find the weight is not coming off. (Most pregnancy weight, around twenty pounds, is typically lost within the first month of giving birth.) Or, you're not such a new mom and still find the extra weight on your frame after a year or more. Friends are telling you, "Once you've given birth, your figure will never be the same." Some women think that pregnancy alters their body; their abdominals will be irreversibly stretched and their hips forever widened. But according to research and experts, that is *not* true. There is no reason you can't get back to your prebaby shape and even look better than before, no matter how long ago you had your baby.

There are many factors that influence weight loss, such as genetics and how in shape you were before you had your baby. Another factor is age. The younger you are, the easier it will be to lose the weight. As you get older, your metabolism slows down and you need fewer calories to sustain the same body weight. Even if you don't exercise less, you can still gain weight. Starting at age twenty-five, your metabolism slows each decade by about 2 percent; assuming your eating and exercise habits remain the same, you could gain a little under a pound a year, or about eight pounds over a ten-year period. Studies indicate that extra pounds are not inevitable after pregnancy, and postpartum weight retention is not necessarily linked to pregnancy itself. Parenting can make you gain weight. Having less time to yourself to go to the gym and exercise coupled with poor diet are the major reasons for weight gain.

Increasing your metabolic rate can be accomplished through exercise and strength training. Muscle is active tissue that consumes calories. The more you build muscle, the more calories you will burn. Studies have shown that strength training can counteract age-related muscle loss and weight gain.

The exercises that I describe here are designed to be more intense than the previous ones and are geared to build muscle. They also center on core and stability strength to improve your abdominals and lower back.

Focus on getting in three thirty-minute workouts per week. Make sure you include exercises for the upper and lower body. Leave your abdominals for last; tired abs will affect the remainder of your workout.

Most important: it took you nine months to put on the weight; give yourself a year to take off the weight. It *will* come off, with commitment and dedication.

CARDIOVASCULAR GOAL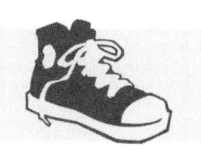

Continue with your cross-training program. Continue to monitor your heart rate. Your goal should be to exercise for twenty to thirty minutes at your target heart rate level. Breaking up your cardiovascular program into two or three ten-minute sessions a day is okay; the goal is to make sure you get it in three times per week. Just because it's been six weeks since your baby was born doesn't mean you're up to your pre-pregnancy work-out. Listen to your body. If you feel tired, weak, or breathless during a workout, stop for the day. When your baby is approximately six months of age and has better head control and strength, take him out for a jog or cycle in a jog stroller or bike trailer.

RECOMMENDED STRENGTH-TRAINING EXERCISES

The following exercises are more advanced and should be done only if you've mastered the exercises in weeks one through five. They should be done in addition to the previous exercises. A good rule of thumb is to do two exercises for each muscle group, every other day. Try to do 2 sets of 8 to 12 repetitions each set.

UPPER BODY

PUSH-UPS ON BALL

(Targets all areas of the upper body)
Get into a push-up position with an exercise ball under your knees. Keep your back straight, hands shoulder width apart, thumbs pointing toward each other. Keep your elbows straight but not locked and your abdominal muscles contracted so that your midsection is stabilized throughout the exercise. Slowly bend your elbows and lower your chest to the ground. When you are two inches from the ground, slowly return to the starting position.

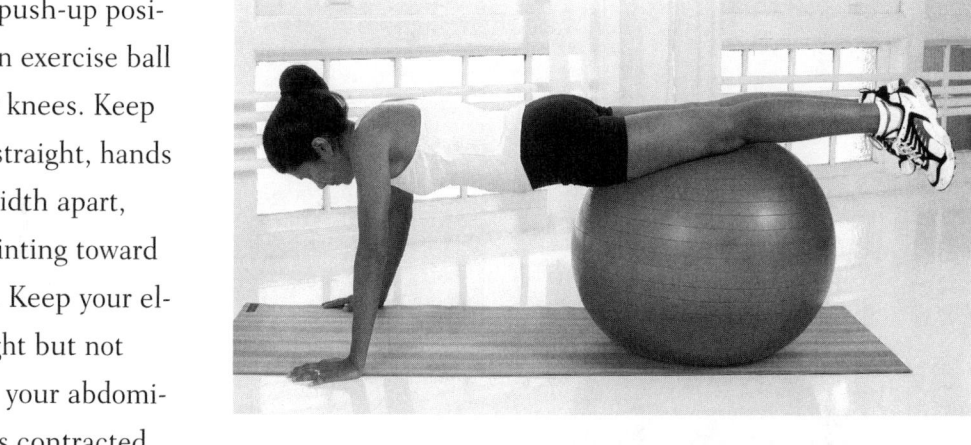

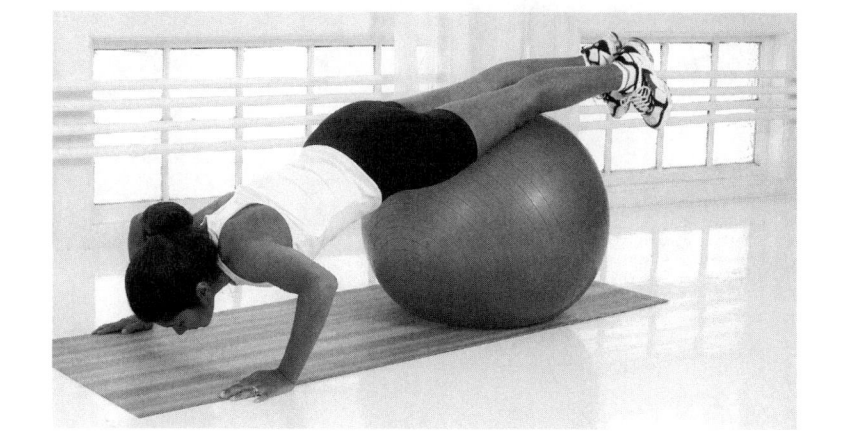

CHEST PRESS ON BALL

(Targets pectoralis major, fronts of deltoids, and triceps)
Lie back on a ball so your head and neck are stabilized. Keep the abdominals and buttocks tight. Push your hips up toward the ceiling. Take a dumbbell in each hand and hold them above you, with your palms facing out. Keep the dumbbells shoulder width apart. Don't allow your hips to drop toward the floor. Slowly lower the dumbbells toward your armpits. Pause, then raise them back to the starting position.

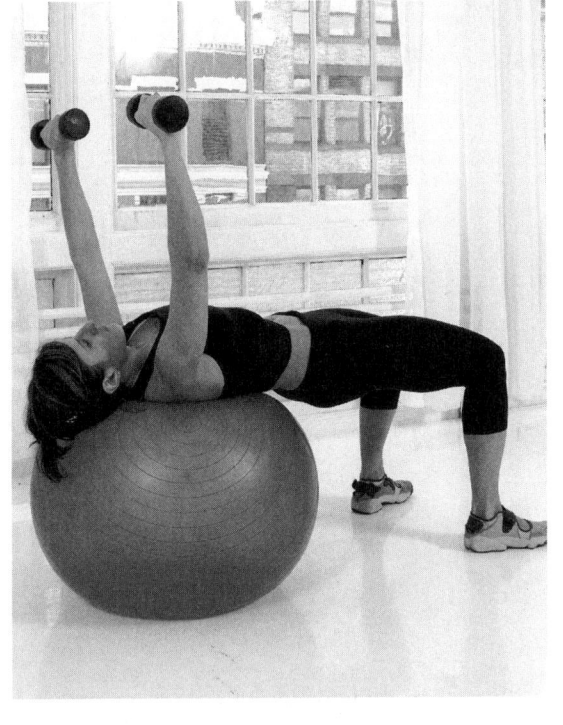
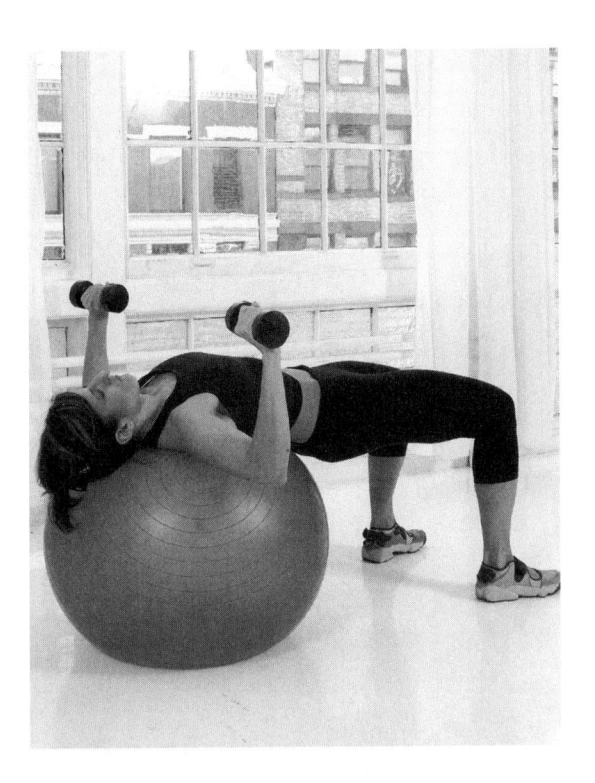

OVERHEAD PRESS

(Targets deltoids, lower back, abdominals)

Sit on a ball, your feet flat on the floor. Maintain a flat back by keeping your abdominals tight. Hold two dumbbells in front of your shoulders, palms facing out. Look straight ahead, keeping your head steady. Extend your arms and lift the dumbbells over your head. The dumbbells should nearly touch each other at the extension. Pause, then lower the weights to the starting position. Make sure not to lock your elbows and not to arch your lower back.

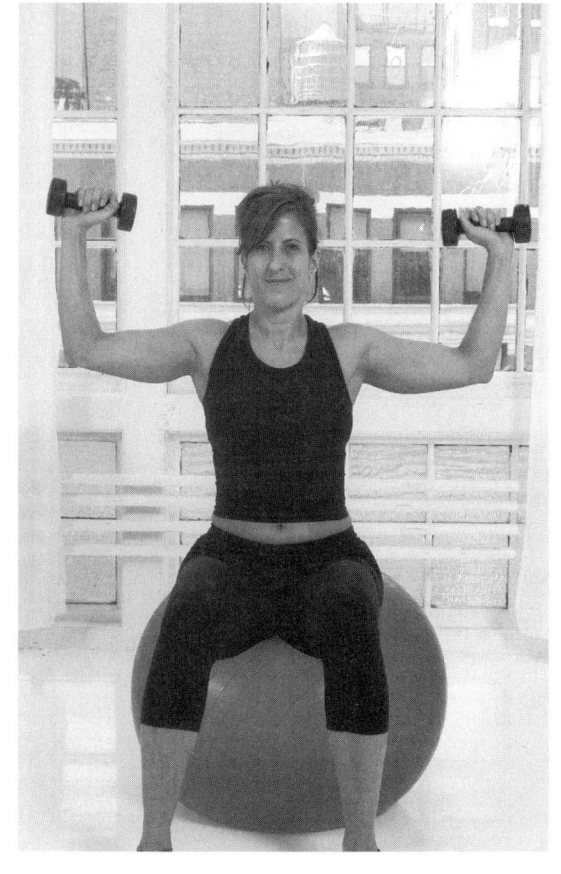
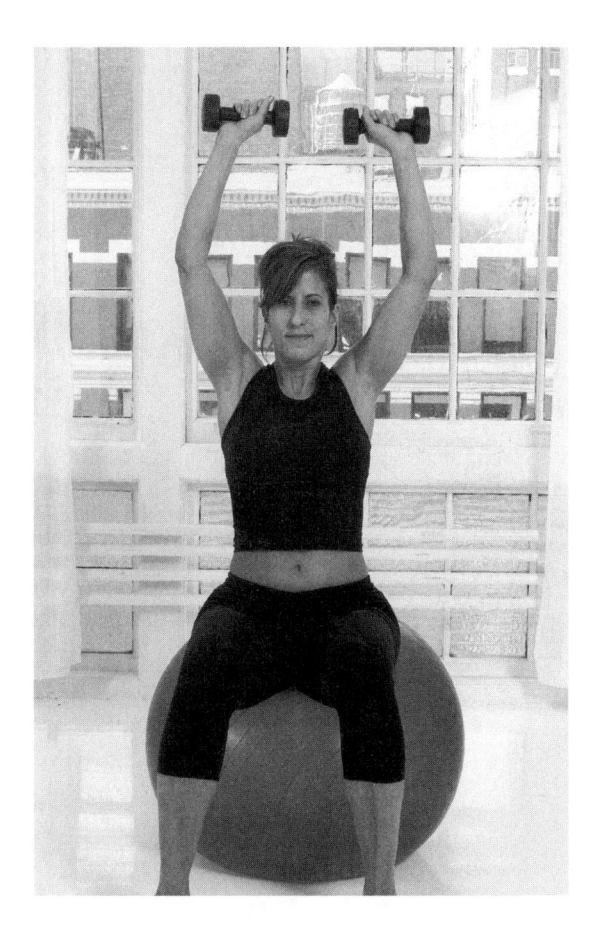

ALTERNATING BICEPS CURLS ON BALL

(Targets biceps, improves core strength and stability)

Sit on a ball with your feet flat on the floor, shoulder width apart. Hold a dumbbell in each hand, palms facing in. Slowly bend your left elbow upward, rotating the forearm so your palm faces your shoulder. Pause, then lower to the starting position. Repeat with the other arm.

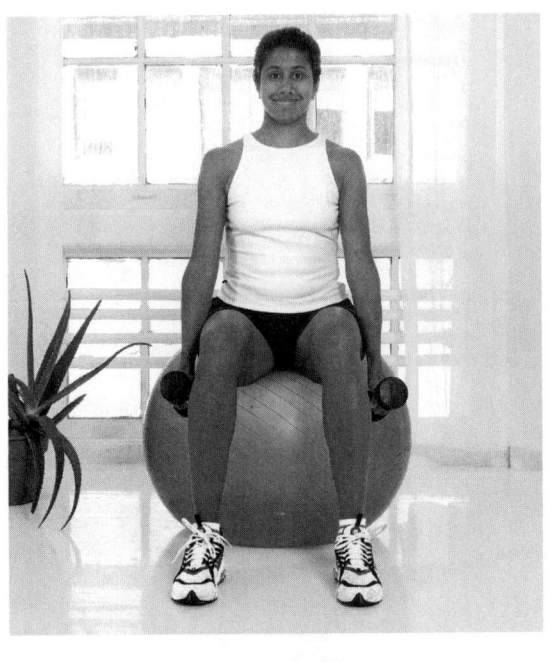 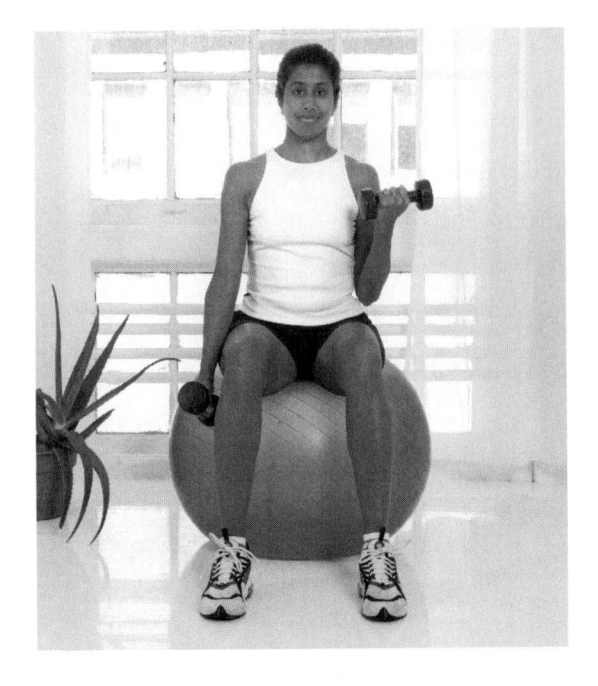

TRICEPS DIPS

(Targets triceps)

Sit on a sturdy bench or chair, your hands gripping the front edge of the seat. Your legs should be bent with your feet flat on floor. With your legs together, move forward until your hips and buttocks are off the seat. Slowly lower your buttocks toward the floor, keeping your abdominals tight and your elbows pointing behind you. Don't let your elbows flare out to the sides. Don't go below a 90-degree angle. Slowly raise your body back to the starting position. Do one set of 8 to 10 repetitions.

SIDE PLANK SHOULDER RAISE

(Targets deltoids, latissimus dorsi, trapezius, abdominals, and back)

Place your left hand on the floor, so it is in direct line with your left shoulder, then extend both of your legs sideways, placing your left foot behind the right.* Tighten your abs so your body forms a straight line from head to feet. Hold a dumbbell in your right hand, arm extended, palm facing in, resting on your hip. Keep your head steady, looking forward. Lift your right arm up toward ceiling, creating a straight vertical line with your supporting arm. Slowly lower to the starting position. After you've completed one set, switch sides.

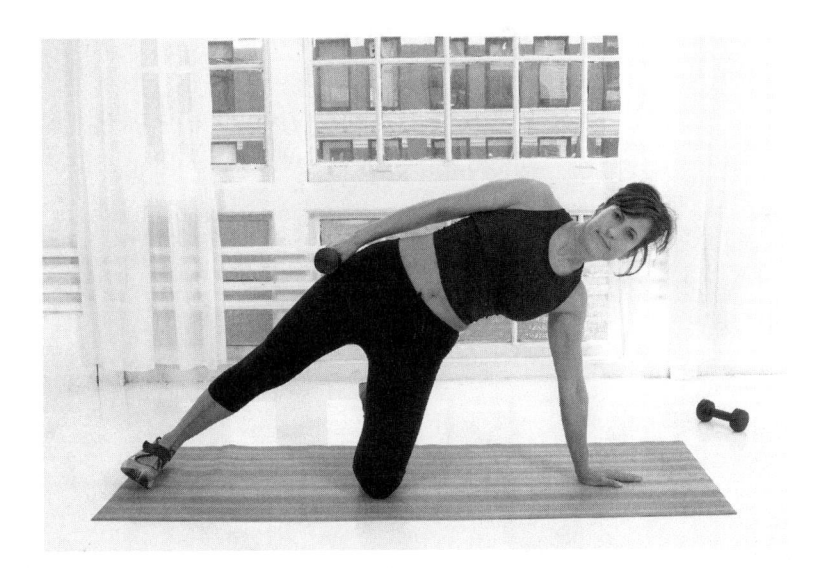

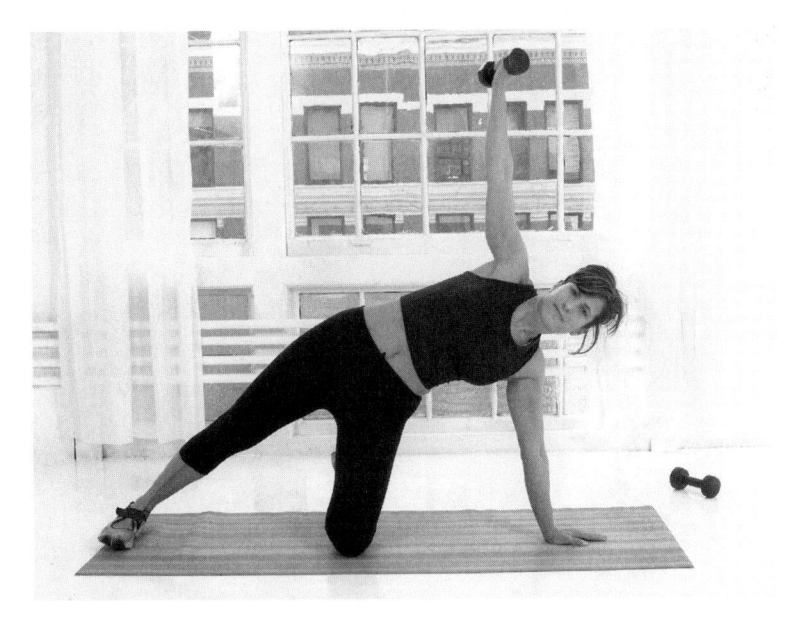

*If you find extending both legs is too difficult, extend only your right leg and place your left knee on the ground.

LOWER BODY

SQUATS WITH BALL

(Targets the quadriceps and buttocks)
Standing, with your feet shoulder width apart, place a ball between the middle of your back and a wall. Keeping your back straight and abdominals tight, slowly bend your knees and squat to a 90-degree angle. Your knees should stay over your toes. Pushing through your heels, return to the starting position.

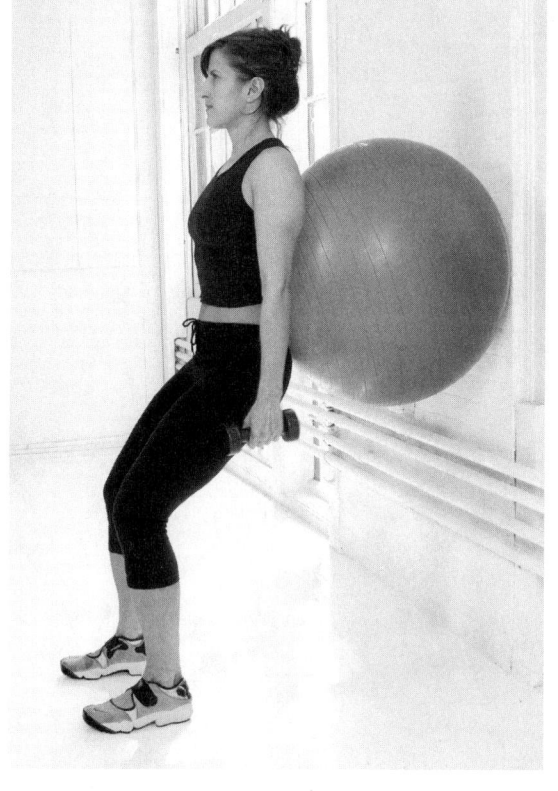 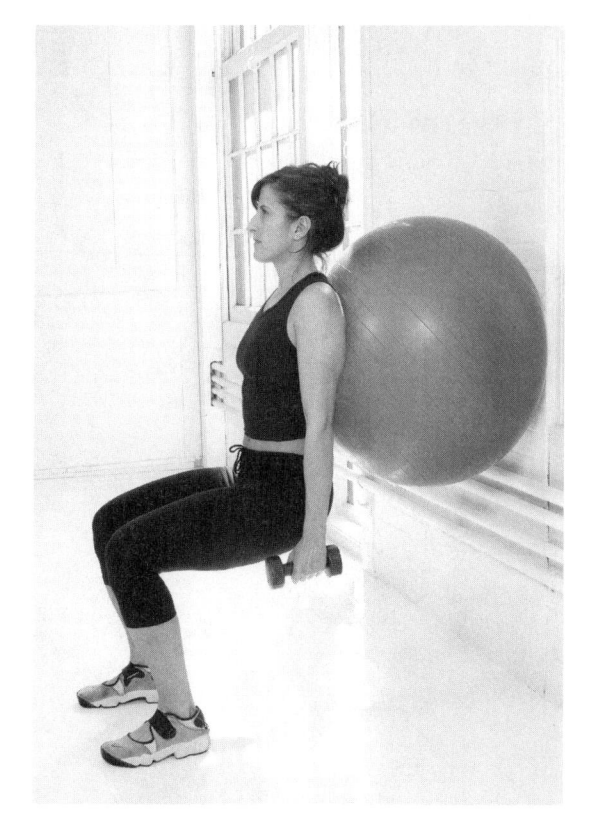

FRONT LUNGE WITH A TWIST

(Targets quadriceps, hamstrings, buttocks, and calves)

Stand with your feet hip width apart. Hold a dumbbell in front of you with
both hands, arms extended at chest height. Contract your abdominals and
take a large step with your left foot, bending your knees so your left knee
aligns with your ankle and does not go past your toes. Bend your right knee
so it nearly touches the ground. Hold the lunge and rotate your torso, arms
still extended, as far as you can go to the left without turning your hips. Rotate back to the starting position and repeat. Do one set of 8 to 10 repetitions.

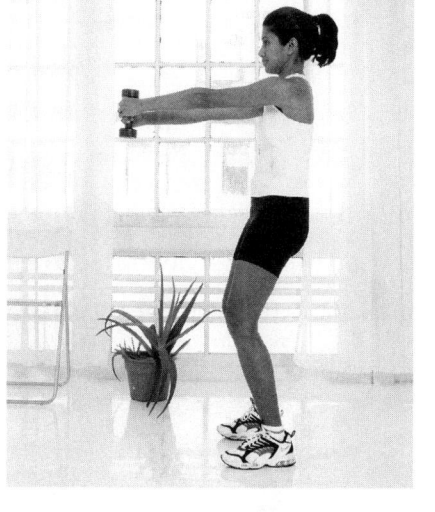
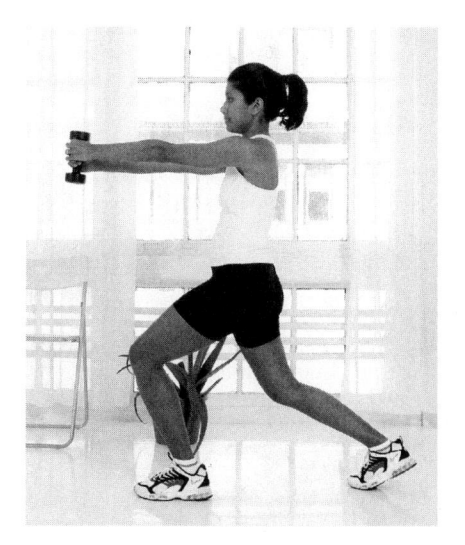
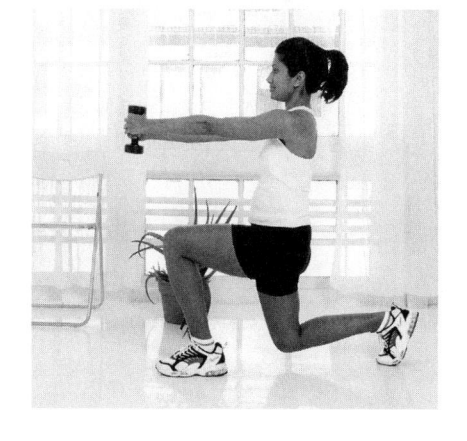
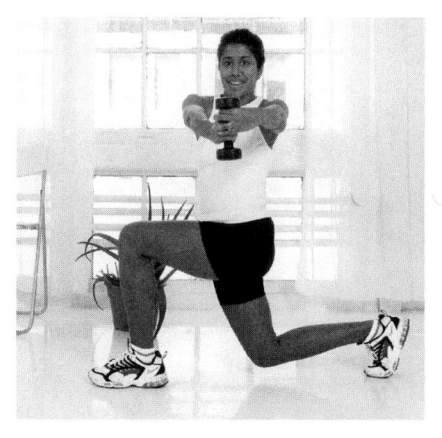

ABDOMINALS/LOWER BACK

BALL ROLL

Kneeling, place your forearms and hands (clasped together) on a ball. Your hips should be in line with your knees. Keeping your abdominals tight and back straight, roll forward about 6 to 8 inches or until you feel a tightening in your lower back and abdominals. Pause, then slowly roll back to the starting position. Start with one set of 8 to 10 repetitions.

SITTING OBLIQUES

Sit on a ball and roll forward until the ball is under your lower back. Place your hands behind your head, your thumbs below your earlobes. Raise the upper body toward your knees and over to the left side; at the same time lift the left leg toward the right shoulder. Pause, then return to the starting position. Repeat on the other side.

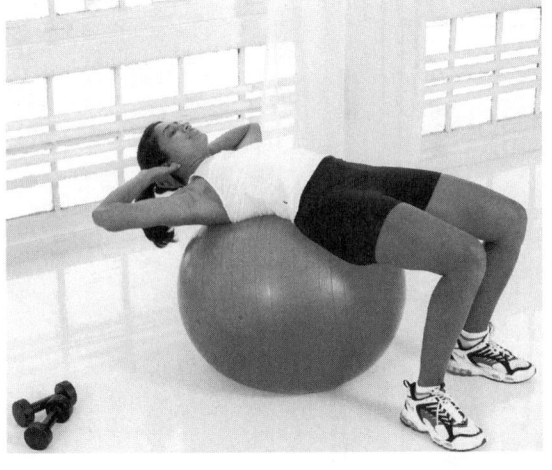
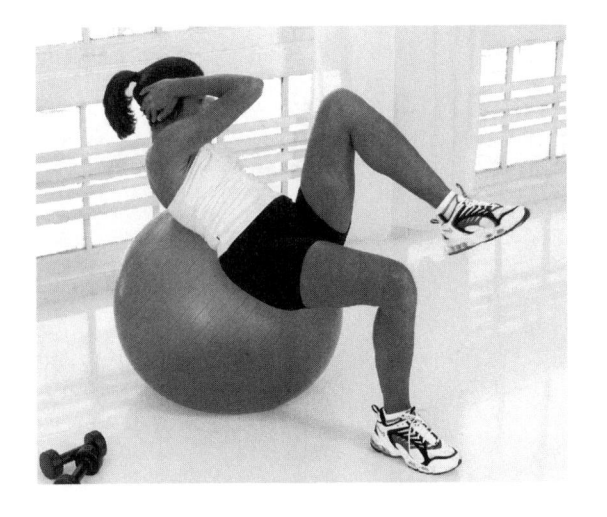

LOWER BACK

LOWER BACK EXTENSION

Lie with the ball under your pelvis and stomach. Place your feet and toes on the floor and your hands on the ball shoulder width apart. Tighten your abdominals and slowly push your chest up and your pelvis into the ball. Straighten your arms as you extend your spine away from the ball. Keep looking straight ahead; don't lean your head backward. Don't overextend your lower back. Pause, then lower to the starting position.

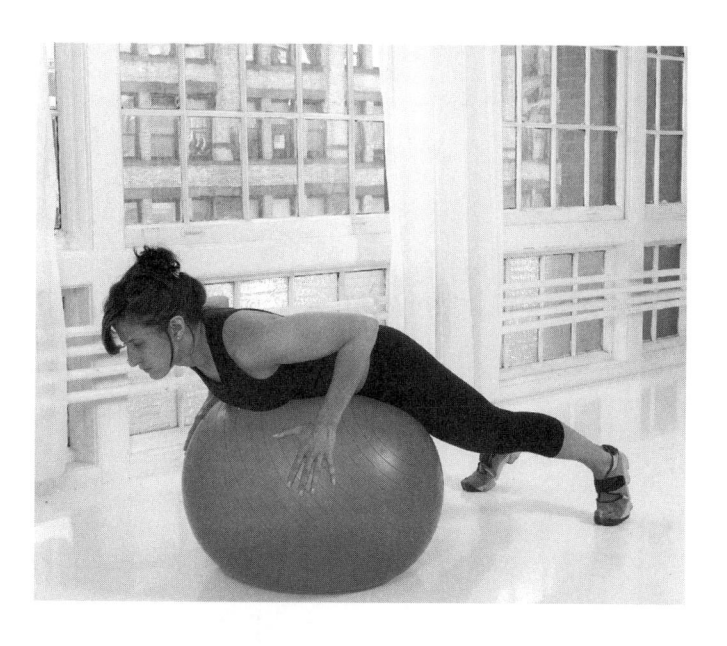

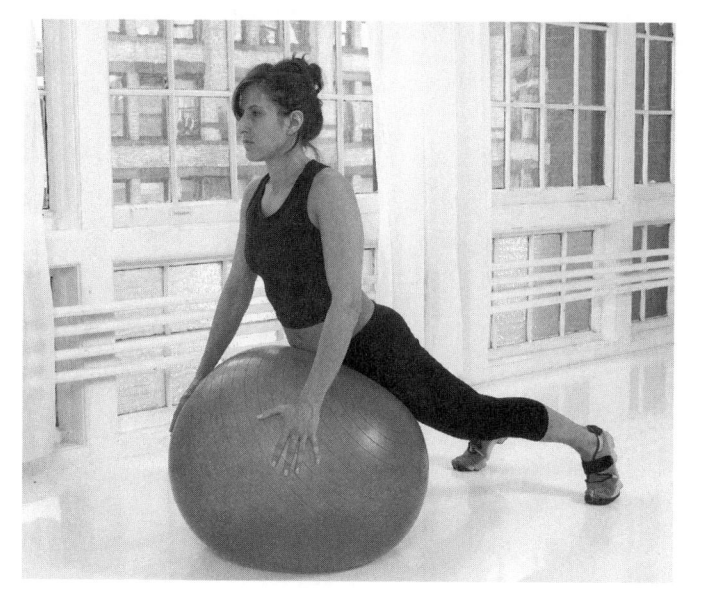

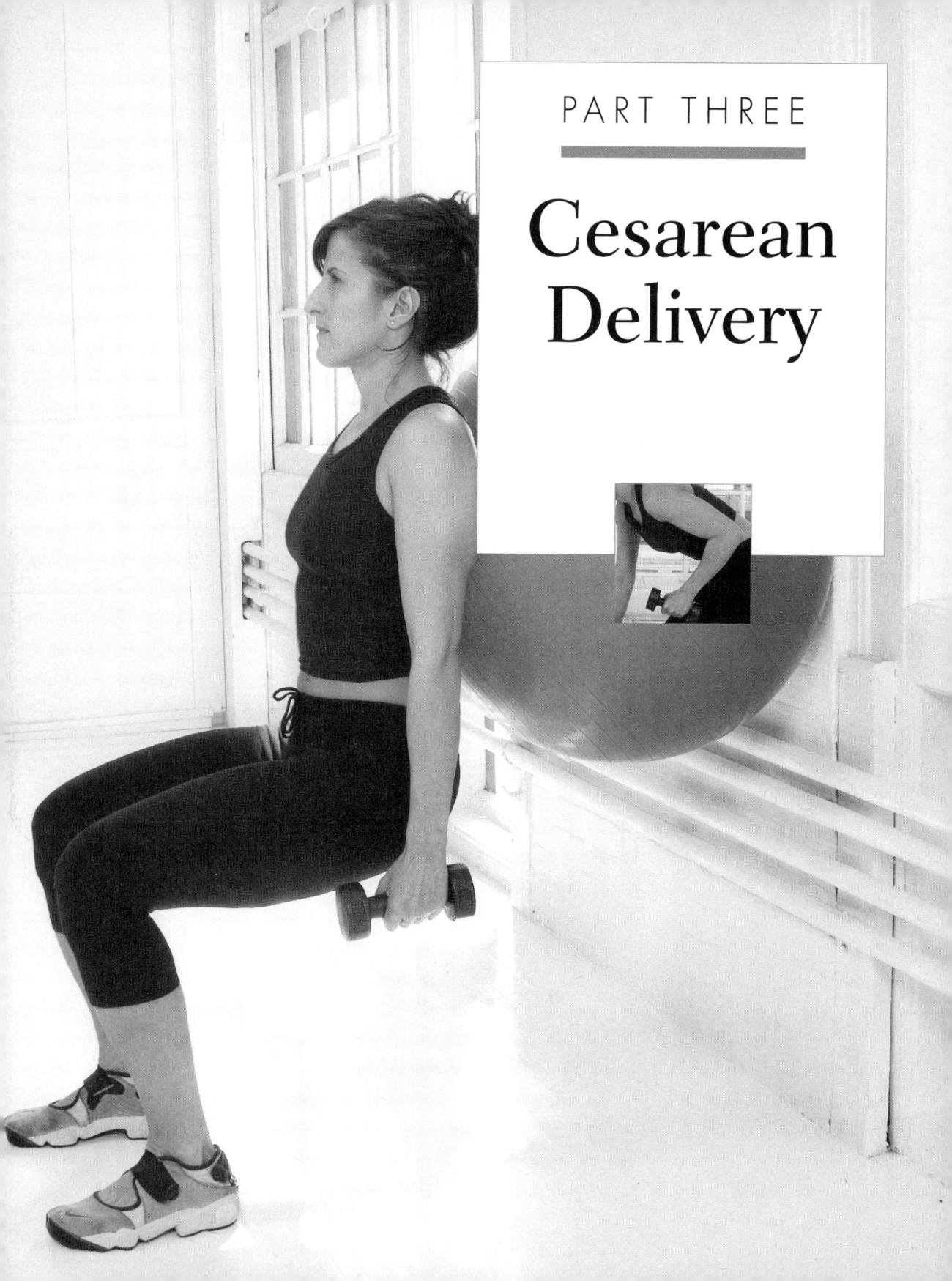

PART THREE

Cesarean Delivery

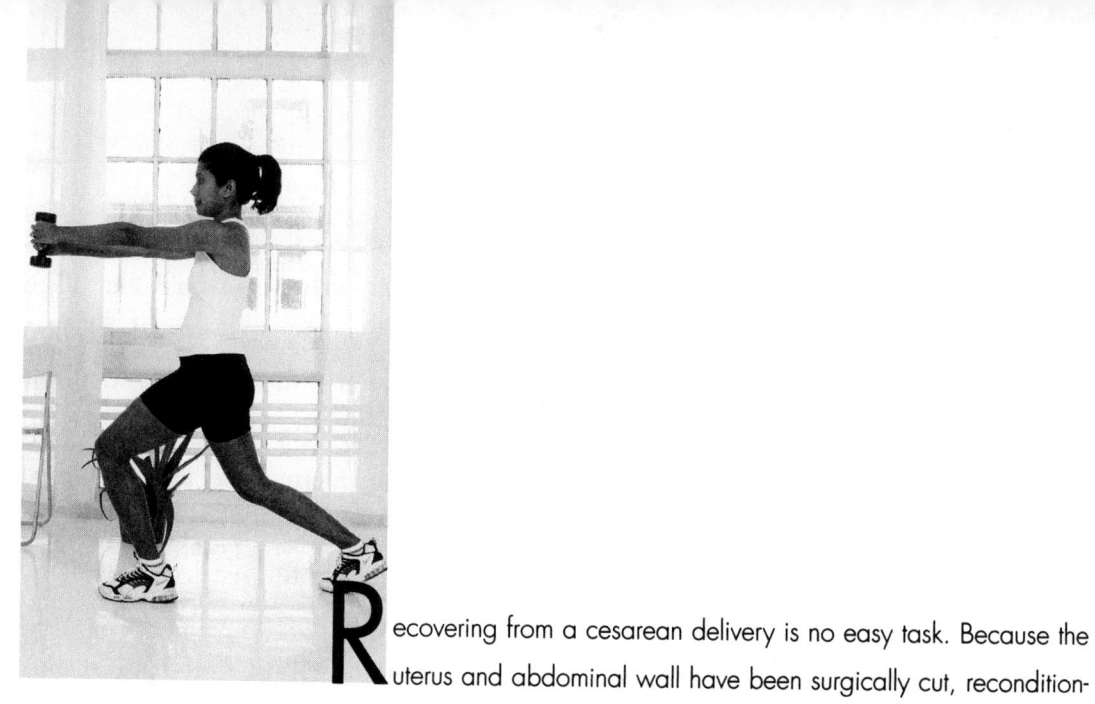

Recovering from a cesarean delivery is no easy task. Because the uterus and abdominal wall have been surgically cut, reconditioning must wait until the sutures have healed, a process that may take up to six weeks. Then, however, you do not have to worry about injuring the incision sites during exercise. Scar tissue is very strong. You can begin postpartum exercises as if you'd had a vaginal delivery. And because the baby has not passed through the birth canal, some of the problems associated with the pelvic floor (tearing, episiotomy pain, anal sphincter stretching or tearing) are much less severe or are absent entirely.

Before your baby arrives you'll most likely think that once you get home, you will be able to do it all. However, you'll soon find out that the housework and all of the other chores will have to be put on hold. You will be too exhausted from 2 A.M. feedings to lift a finger, let alone wash the dishes. Let your family, husband, or partner help you out those first few weeks. If you are bottle-feeding, let him participate in the ritual. Let him change diapers and take your place on a few of the early morning feedings. The more you let others do during the recovery period, the faster you'll recuperate.

Avoid using your tummy muscles the first few weeks. You may be able to do easy abdominal exercises ten to fourteen days after your C-section, but do them only if you feel up to it. If you find that you can't get in and out of bed without pain, try sleeping on a couch that you can easily lift yourself off of, or place a chair near the edge of the bed. Pulling up with assistance will make this task easier. Do not lift anything heavy the first three to four weeks after a cesarean section.

A common question I hear from women who've had a C-section is, "When can I start doing sit-ups to flatten my tummy?" Generally, you can start four to six weeks after delivery. However, everyone is different. Some women may be able to do easy curl-ups ten days postpartum. Make sure you get the approval from your doctor before starting any form of exercise after a C-section.

I remind all of my clients that as they set out to flatten their tummies, to keep in mind that there is no such thing as "spot reduction." Doing three hundred sit-ups a day is not going to give you those six-pack abs. The only way to meet your goal is through a combination of cardiovascular exercise, good nutrition, and strength training. Crunches, sit-ups, and other abdominal exercises are important, but if you perform just those you'll only strengthen the muscles below the extra fat, and you'll probably not see improvement on the outside.

Multiple C-Sections

It was once widely accepted that most women who gave birth via C-section had to have a repeat cesarean section for each subsequent delivery. The traditional method of doing a C-section was to make a vertical incision in the upper part of the uterus. Incisions like this are more likely to rupture when labor begins, leading to bleeding that can put both the mother and child at risk. However, a woman who has had a transverse incision (as opposed to the classical vertical incision) is a better candidate for a vaginal birth after cesarean (VBAC). This is because the incision cuts through the lower part of the uterus, which has fewer muscles and blood vessels, lowering the chances of bleeding due to uterine rupture. The present practice for women who have had previous cesarean sections with a low transverse incision is to give them a trial labor with the goal of a vaginal birth. However, doctors are prepared to perform an emergency cesarean should the need arise.

During the 1970s and early 1980s, cesarean deliveries increased from about 5 percent to nearly 25 percent of all births. Since then, public health experts have expressed concern that cesarean delivery has been overused by obstetricians. Today, doctors have more guidelines to help them determine when it is necessary.

Why the concern about cesarean birth? While the infant usually benefits from a C-section, the mother is usually more at risk. There is a higher rate of complications and the postpartum recovery is longer.

After a routine cesarean delivery, most women are encouraged to begin walking short distances within twenty-four hours. Walking can help relieve gas buildup in the abdomen. It is usually very uncomfortable to begin walking, but the pain will decrease in the days after the delivery. After about four weeks, more vigorous exercise is encouraged; however, it isn't unusual to have occasional pains in the C-section area during the first year after surgery.

After a C-section, you may find yourself leaning forward and toward the side of your incision. As you walk, support the incision with your hands and try to keep your back straight. Keep your head and shoulders back and over your hips. Try to keep your abdominal muscles tightened. This will not pull apart your incision.

Minimize stair-climbing during the first few weeks. If you must, go up and down stairs slowly, one step at a time, to avoid becoming tired. Use your thigh and hip muscles to step. Keep your back straight and your weight over your feet. When bending over, keep one foot in front of the other. Bend your knees and lower your trunk. Your legs should take most of the weight. To lift *light* objects, put one foot in front of the other and keep the object close to your body. When reaching, use a stool to avoid overstretching.

Emotional Adjustment

You may find yourself feeling such emotions as anger, relief, resentment, disappointment, and guilt after having a C-section. Some new moms may wish they had had a more active part in the labor. These feelings are quite normal. You may find it helpful to discuss them with your partner and doctor. Find out as much information as you can about your delivery.

The Exercise Plan

Ask your doctor to review with you the value of exercise, deep breathing, and good body mechanics for recovery after your cesarean section.

Although rigorous exercise is not advised by this author or any medical professional, the following recommendations are the key to successful C-section rehabilitation. You will progress in the exercises the first five or six days or until you can safely demonstrate the routine below. Again, DO NOT START ANY EXERCISE PROGRAM UNLESS ADVISED BY YOUR DOCTOR.

Day 1

Doing deep-breathing techniques is important the first day after a cesarean section. If general anesthesia was used, secretions may pool in your lungs. Frequent deep breaths are necessary so that your lungs completely fill with air.

Try to do each of these breathing techniques:

BREATHING WITH THE DIAPHRAGM

Support your incision with your hand or a pillow. Take deep breaths so it feels as though you are filling your stomach with air. Don't worry about your incision opening.

MIDCHEST EXPANSION

Place your hands on your lower ribs. Take a deep breath and try to expand your lungs in the area under your hands.

UPPER CHEST EXPANSION

Place your hands over your upper chest, breathe in deeply and direct the air through your chest.

103

DEEP BREATHING

Support your incision with your hand or a pillow. Breathe in through your nose, exhale out of your mouth.

PELVIC-FLOOR EXERCISES

(also known as Kegel exercises [see pages 46–47]

1. Tighten and relax the muscles around your birth canal. Take deep breaths in as you are doing this.

2. Tighten the muscles of your bottom and at the same time squeeze your thighs together. Tighten the muscles around your birth canal as if to stop the flow of urine. Hold 5 to 8 seconds.

ANKLE CIRCLES

Make ten circles with your ankles, clockwise then counterclockwise.

LEG BRACING

Cross your ankles and straighten your legs. Tighten your thighs and squeeze your buttocks together. Hold for 5 to 10 seconds. Repeat 3 to 5 times.

WALKING

If you feel up to it, a short walk is recommended twenty-four hours after having a C-section. Make sure you have someone assisting you.

Days 2 and 3

Repeat all of the breathing exercises, Kegels, and lower-body exercises from day 1. Keep taking short walks as well, but don't overdo it.

PELVIC-TILT EXERCISES

Lie on your back with your knees bent and feet flat on the floor. Try to push your lower back into the floor, keeping your butt tight.

LEG SLIDES

Lying on your back, bend your right leg, keeping your foot flat on the floor. Keep your left leg extended on the floor. Pushing your lower back into the floor, slide your left heel up and down, keeping your right leg bent. Do 8 to 10 times; repeat with the right leg.

MODIFIED BRIDGE

Lying with your legs extended on the floor, lift your left hip slightly up and down 8 to 10 times. Repeat with the right side.

Days 4 Through 9

At this point, hopefully, you are moving around without too much pain. Continue with the exercises from days 2 and 3 and slowly increase the duration of your short walks. Listen to your body; if you start to tire or feel discomfort, take it easy.

HEAD SIT-UPS

Lying on your back, bend your legs slightly, keeping your feet flat on the floor. Cross your hands over your stomach and pull your abdominal muscles together with your hands. Lift your head off the floor, leading with your chin. Do not bring your chin to your chest, as it will strain your neck. Hold for 3 seconds, repeat. Try to do 5 to 8 repetitions.

ROCKERS

Lying on your back, bend your legs slightly, keeping your feet flat on the floor. Extend your arms out to either side, palms down and shoulders flat. Keeping your knees together, first roll them to the right, then to the left. If you can touch the ground on each side, great, but if you feel discomfort, don't try to force your knees all the way down. Repeat 8 to 10 times.

Day 10 and Beyond

Continue with all of the exercises from day 1 and add the following:

PELVIC TILT

On your hands and knees, pull your abdominals in through your belly button. Arch your back toward the ceiling as high as you can, tucking your pelvis, and hold for 5 to 8 seconds. Repeat 8 to 10 times.

ABDOMINAL EXERCISES

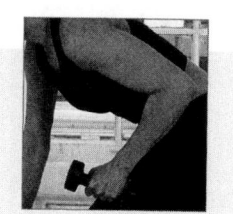

Before doing any of the abdominal exercises, make sure you don't have a diastasis (see page 58 for a full description of a diastasis). If you do have a diastasis, you need to vary the abdominal exercises to give more support to the area. For both of the abdominal exercises, use your hands and arms to support your stomach muscles. Cross your hands over your abdomen, and pull the abdominal muscles together. Or put a towel around your waist, crisscrossing the ends in front and pulling them together.

Do one of the following abdominal exercises. If you find pillow sit-ups too easy, try the curl-ups.

Pillow Sit-ups

Place pillows behind your lower back so you're in a sitting position, leaning back slightly. Bend your knees, feet flat on the floor. Tuck your chin, exhale, and reach toward the sides of your knees with your hands. Hold for 2 to 3 seconds, then return to the starting position. Repeat 6 to 10 times.

Curl-ups

Lying on your back with your knees bent and feet flat on the floor, place your hands behind your head, thumbs underneath your earlobes, elbows out. Lift your head off the floor, leading with your chin. Don't pull your head with your hands; focus on using the abdominal muscles. Breathe out on the way up, inhale on the way down. Repeat 5 to 10 times.

You should be walking easily at this point. Continue with daily walking.

Communicate with your doctor before you go ahead with more strenuous exercise. Once you have the okay, usually 4 to 6 weeks after delivery, follow the exercise program described in Part Two.

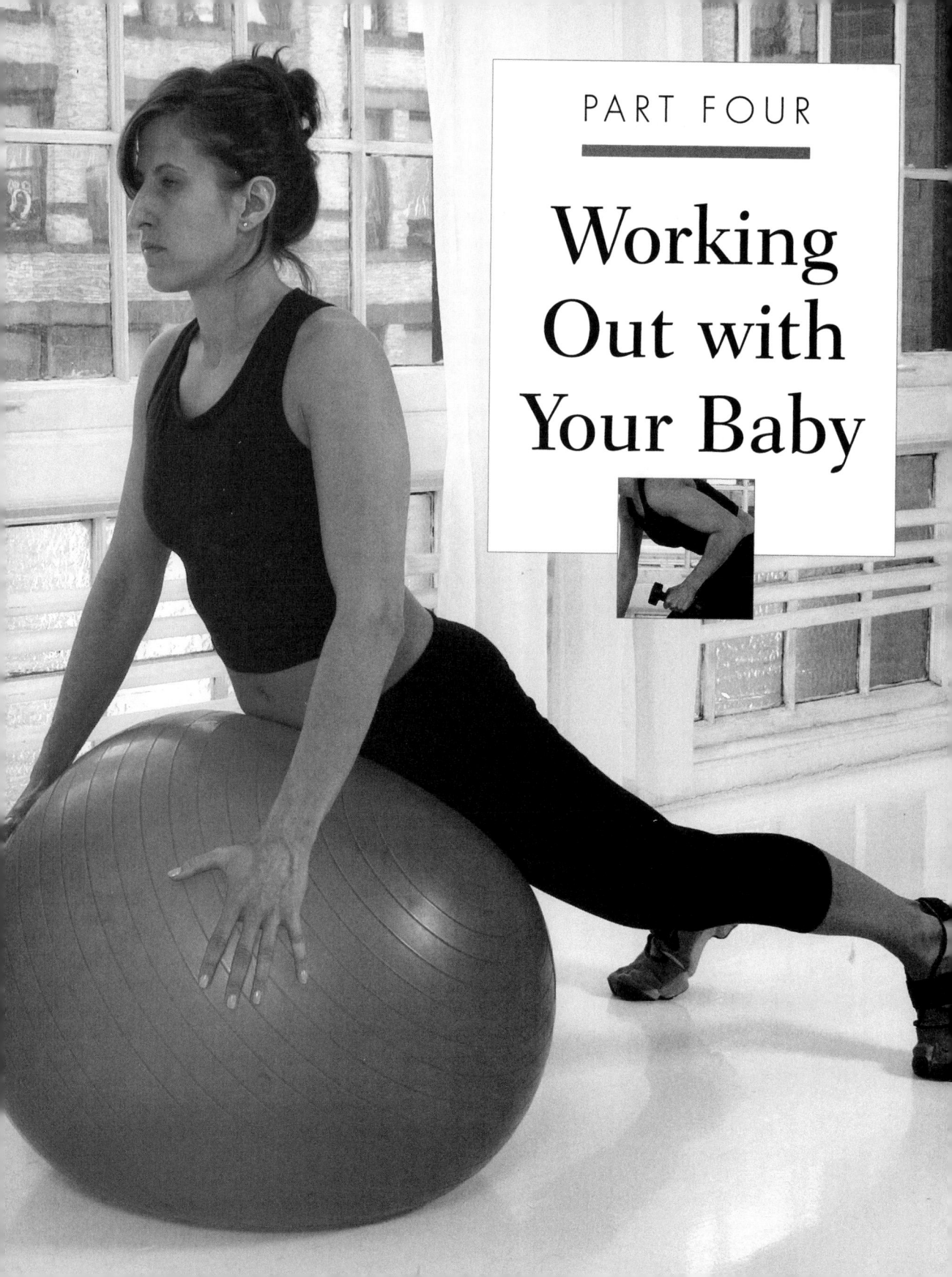

PART FOUR

Working Out with Your Baby

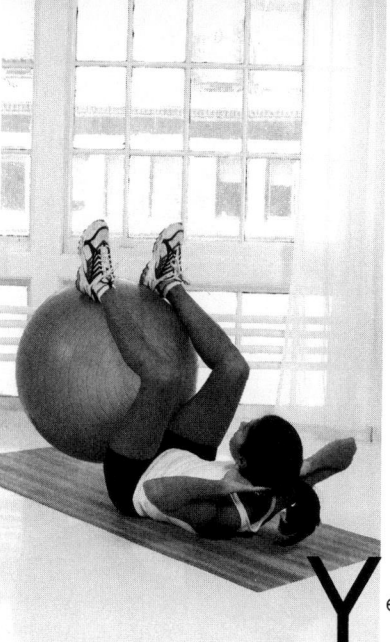

Yes, believe it or not, you can get your body back by working out with your baby. When your baby is still tiny, a baby sling and/or carrier work well for walking. When you are physically up for running, a baby jogger is a great tool for bringing your baby along. However, make sure you wait a few months to let the developing muscles of your baby's back and neck get stronger.

I've outlined some fun, easy, strength-training exercises that are safe for both you and baby. Give them a try!

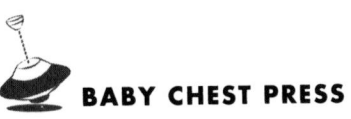

BABY CHEST PRESS

Lying on your back on a carpeted floor or mat, hold your baby in both hands and extend your arms straight up. Try not to lock your arms, then slowly lower to the starting position. This exercise is great for strengthening your pectoralis muscles. Do 2 sets of 12 repetitions.

LEG LIFTS WITH BABY

Sitting in a chair, extend your right leg. Place your baby right below your knee, holding its hands. Slowly raise your leg and baby, about 3 to 4 inches, then lower to the starting position. This exercise is great for strengthening your quadriceps muscles. Do each leg twice, 10 to 12 repetitions.

LULLABY LUNGES

Placing your baby in a stroller, grab the handle firmly with your left hand, with the stroller to your left. Your feet should be shoulder width apart and your abdominals tight. With your right foot, take a step forward, bending your right knee directly over your right toes. Slowly lower your body by bending your left knee. Be sure to keep the right knee over the toes when lowering. Just before your left knee touches the ground, slowly push up. Keep your back straight and your shoulders back. At the same time, you should be gently pushing the stroller forward. Then take a step forward with your left foot, repeating the same motion. This exercise is great for strengthening your quadriceps, glutes, and hamstrings. A complete repetition is lunging once with each leg. Try to do 2 sets of 10 to 12 repetitions.

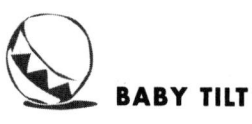 **BABY TILT**

Lie on your back with your baby sitting on top of your stomach. Do a pelvic tilt, using your baby as resistance. Start with one set of 8 to 10 repetitions. Work up to 2 to 3 sets of 10 to 12 repetitions.

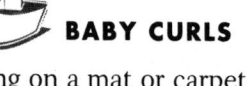 **BABY CURLS**

Lying on a mat or carpeted floor, feet flat on the floor, bend your knees. Place your baby on your stomach, sitting, facing you. Slowly curl up, trying to touch the sides of your knees as you come up. This is great for the abdominals. Start with one set of 8 to 10 repetitions. Work up to 2 to 3 sets of 10 to 12 repetitions.

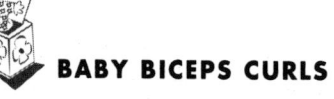 **BABY BICEPS CURLS**

Standing, lift your baby under its arms, supporting its head with your fingers. Keep your elbows tucked into the sides of your body. Slowly curl your baby up and down, keeping your abdominals tight and back straight. Do 2 to 3 sets of 10 to 12 repetitions.

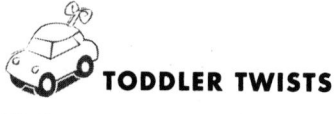 **TODDLER TWISTS**

Sitting on an exercise mat or carpeted floor, cross your legs and hold your baby with both hands. Extend your arms out and gently twist your body to your right, bringing your head and baby to your right side. Pause, then twist to your left side. This exercise targets your abdominal and oblique muscles. Start with one set of 8 to 10 repetitions. Work up to 2 to 3 sets of 10 to 12 repetitions.

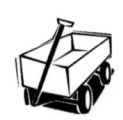

Getting your body back and keeping it is an ongoing process. For most women, the decision to take control of their bodies instead of the other way around is a conscious decision. Fitness is not only physical but mental. Exercising daily will help you look good and give you the stamina and energy that will keep you going throughout the day. Keep exercise a priority!

From a Buff Mom: "I'm happy with the way I look. If you saw me in a bathing suit, you wouldn't necessarily know I'd had two kids!"

ACKNOWLEDGMENTS

There are many wonderful individuals who have worked hard to make this book a reality. So many people helped with such generosity and unfailing support. I am fortunate to have the amazing team at Villard/Random House, especially Bruce Tracy. Your backing, enthusiasm, and encouragement were invaluable. Also, thank you to others at Villard who contributed to the book's completion: Adam Korn, Janet Wygal, and publicist Kate Blum. I'd also like to thank the William Morris Agency, especially the astute and talented Jennifer Rudolph Walsh and Andy McNicol. Your belief in me and support of this project were, at times, almost overwhelming.

I am deeply grateful to the talented people who made enormous contributions to the book. Thank you to Dr. Sarah Kelly for your guidance and wisdom, and to stunning models and moms Anitra Sipp and Darlene Milowski. Thank you to the talented Jack Myers for his superb cover design, and to Patrik Rytikangas for his beautiful photography. A special thank-you to Carol Myers and Barbara Norris at Divine Studio in NYC. Special thanks for the contributions of Virginia Siegrist and Colleen McGowan.

Thank you to my many dear friends and colleagues at Riverdale Country School for their endless support through my book projects, especially Kent Kildahl, John Johnson, David Hooks, Kathy Schoonmaker, Tonia Maschi, Lynn Sorenson, Beth Norman, and the amazing members of the physical education department. I am extremely fortunate to have you, the RCS community, in my life.

My heartfelt thanks goes out to all of those who have supported me through the past two difficult and challenging years of my life. Words cannot express how grateful I am. Thank you to Lauren Van Kirk, Suzanne Borda, Pamela Guyer, Uncle Steve Guyer, Aunt Florence Guyer, Bonnie Eldon, Gretchen Koss, Polly DeFrank, Deborah Larkin, and Sandra DeOvando. You all have become my family.

Finally, one needs a truly beautiful and special environment in which to write. I am fortunate to have found that on the beautiful pink sand beaches of Harbour Island and in the peacefulness and serenity of Claverack, New York. So I thank you, Kate Frucher, for sharing those special memories with me, for sharing those precious parts of life with me. But most of all, thank you for helping me discover how to love deeply and how to truly cherish the value of life.

INDEX

ABOUT THE AUTHOR

SUE FLEMING earned her B.S. and M.S. in
physical education and has been a certified personal trainer for the past ten years. The author of
Buff Brides (now a series on the Discovery Health
Channel) and *Buff Moms-to-Be,* she is currently
the director of physical education at Riverdale
Country School in Riverdale, New York, and
continues to work with private clients. She lives
in Manhattan. Sue Fleming can be reached at
www.buffbrides.com.